PERFECT PARTS

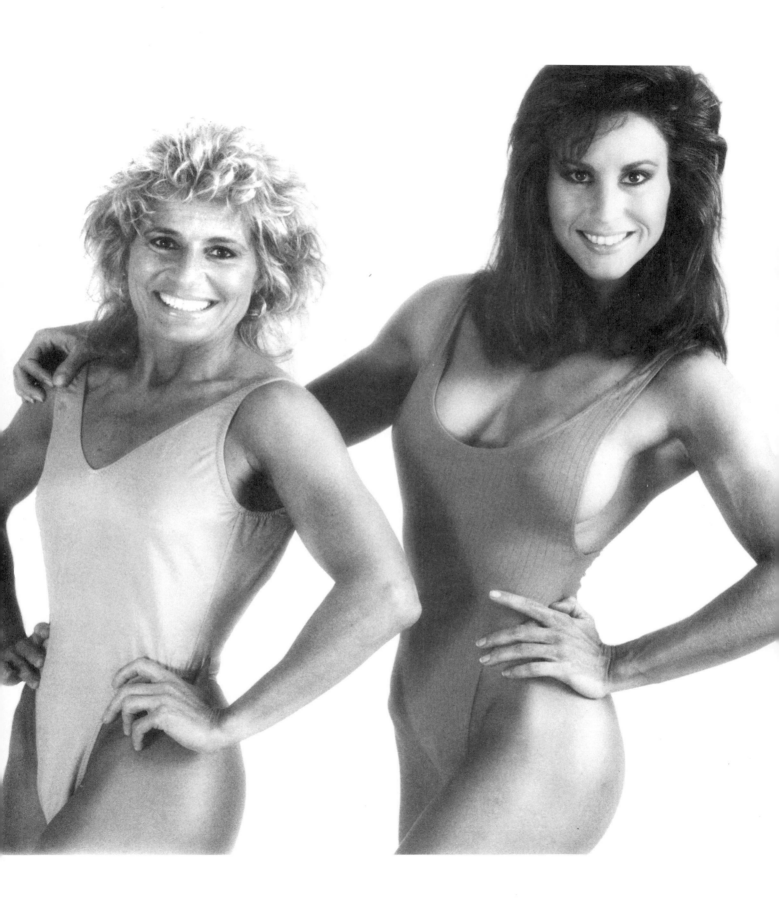

Also by Rachel McLish

FLEX APPEAL

Also by Joyce L. Vedral, Ph.D.

**NOW OR NEVER: The Weight Training Program
That Works Even as You Age**

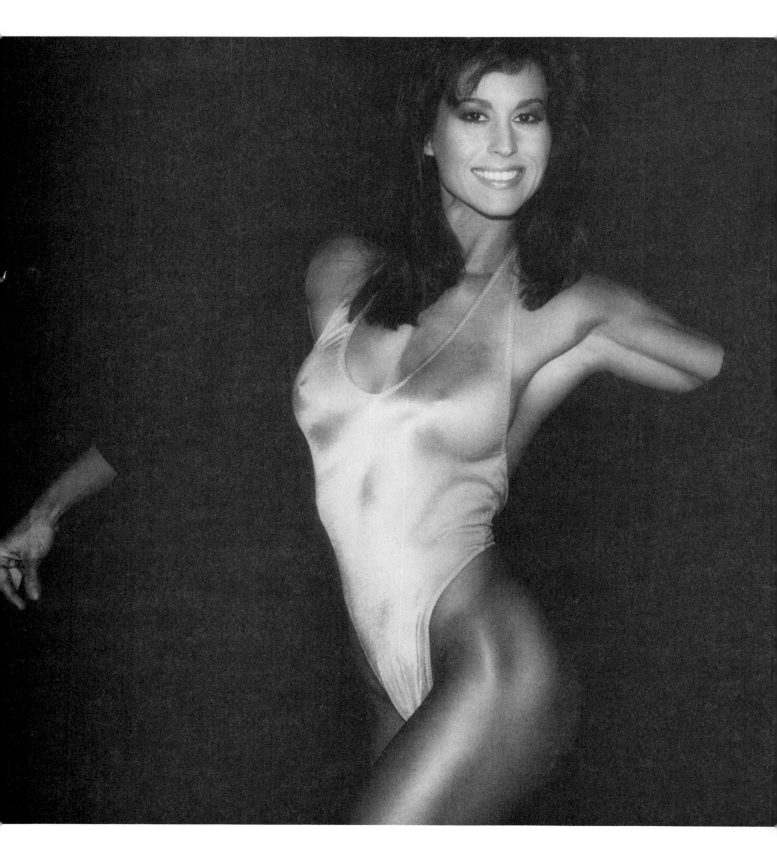

PERFECT PARTS

Rachel McLish

and Joyce L. Vedral, Ph.D.

WARNER BOOKS

A Time Warner Company

Cover photograph © 1987 by Harry Langdon Photography
Cover leotard by Nancy Pollak Bodywear
Cover hair and makeup by Steve Reiley, HMS Bookings
Workout leotards by Danskin, Nancy Pollak Bodywear, and Dedication
Gym photographs shot at World Gym, Venice, California

 A Time Warner Company

Printed in the United States Of America

Designed by Giorgetta Bell McRee
Packaged by Rapid Transcript, a division of March Tenth, Inc.

First Printing: October 1987
20 19 18 17 16 15 14 13 12

Library of Congress Cataloging-in-Publication Data

McLish, Rachel.
    Rachel's perfect parts / Rachel McLish and Joyce L. Vedral.
        p.   cm.
    ISBN 0-446-38534-4 (pbk.) (U.S.A.)   0-446-38535-2 (pbk.) (Canada)
    1. Bodybuilding for women. 2. Exercise for women. I. Vedral,
Joyce L. II. Title.
GV546.6.W64M44   1987
646.7 '5 — dc19   87-15887
                                                                              CIP

To the only perfect person ever—Jesus

Contents

> 1 Day

> second day

Acknowledgments

Thank you, Kathy McBride, for believing in this project and for seeing it through to the end.

Thank you, Paul Goode, for a sensitive, artistic approach to the photographs.

Thank you, Ron Samuels, for your moral support and encouragement and for the use of your lovely home.

Thank you, Joe Gold and Eddie Juliannie, for the use of your wonderful one and only World Gym in Santa Monica, California.

Thank you, my wonderful sister Yolanda, for being patient and supportive through my work on this book—and for taking a lot of the pressure off.

Thank you, Roy Zurkowski, for your continual enthusiasm and your positive attitude.

Thank you, family and friends, for your love, affection, and support every step of the way. (And that includes you, Sandra Lopez.)

Thank you, Joyce Vedral, for your hard work and for understanding that I'm an imperfect perfectionist.

Thank you, Bob Oskam, for your talented and sensitive editing.

Thank you, Joann Davis, for your wisdom in handling every possible problem.

Thank you, my wonderful sister Barbara Vale, for your continual faith and moral support.

Thank you, too, Martha Yellin, my terrific mom, for always being there.

Thank you, Rachel McLish, for being a true friend.

Thank you, God, for Your continual guidance throughout this project. Without You we couldn't have done it.

PERFECT
PARTS

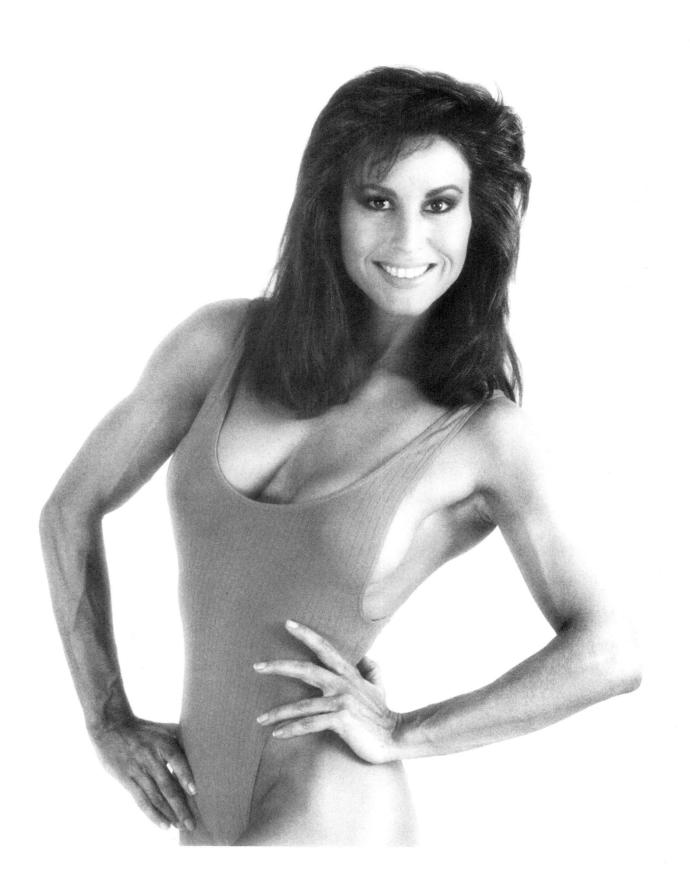

1

The Good News: You <u>Can</u> Spot Change

For years women have been told that it is impossible to spot reduce. And that's true. You can't spot *reduce*, but you can spot *change* (get rid of ugly fat and replace it with firm, sexy muscle) by working with weights the right way. You don't have to work your entire body if you don't want to. You can concentrate just on the body part you want to change: sagging breasts, drooping triceps, broadening buttocks, pencil-thin arms—whatever you want to change—by investing only fifteen minutes two or three times a week per body part. For example, if your goal is only to lift and reshape your sagging buttocks, all you have to do is work out your buttocks area three times a week for fifteen minutes. That's it. Of course, you may get carried away once you see the wonderful results and want to work on your entire body. That will be your choice, however.

HOW IS SPOT CHANGE POSSIBLE?

When you work on a given body part with weights, following the routines given in this book, you stimulate the muscles in that area by increasing the blood flow to them and demanding that they respond. They firm up—lose their flabby quality—and begin to grow. At the same time, you burn fat from that particular area. For example, when you do twenty-five sit-ups, rest, then do another twenty-five sit-ups and so on, you burn

1

intramuscular fat that contributes to shapeless sag at the same time that you build a tight girdle of shapely muscles. Eventually your stomach flattens, becoming sensual as muscles begin to develop in just the right places.

The idea of working one body part at a time is not new. Everyone who works out in a gym works one body part at a time. Gyms have machines specially designed to stimulate *not* the whole body but specific body parts or muscle groups. There are calf machines, biceps machines, shoulder machines, and so on. If the whole body could be developed with a single set of exercises, it would save gym owners a fortune. All they would have to do would be to invest in one big machine. Think of how easy it would be for everyone to get in shape.

All champion bodybuilders work one body part at a time. They do a series of exercises for the chest, then a group of exercises for the shoulders, then another group of exercises for the thighs, and so on. The developed parts combine into a developed whole. In fact, if a bodybuilder neglects to work on a particular body part, that body part will stand out as an eyesore. It will look underdeveloped next to the other, more developed body parts. I've seen this happen with bodybuilders who neglect working on their calves or abdominals. They often lose contests because the eyes of the judges go straight to the untrained body part.

I have seen how the body develops by working specific muscle groups in isolation in my own experience. At the age of seven I began ballet lessons, and I continued to dance for ten years. By the time I was seventeen my legs were highly developed, while the rest of my body was underdeveloped. Observe the forearms of tennis players—especially the hitting forearm. Notice the calves of runners, the arms and shoulders of swimmers, and the necks and backs of wrestlers. Each of these is a living example of spot body development by regular stimulation of particular areas.

WHY DIETING ALONE CANNOT RESHAPE BODY PARTS

Why do people say, "It's impossible to spot reduce"? They say this because it *is* in fact impossible when using the conventional method women turn to in order to change the shape of their bodies, dieting.

For years, women have been under the false impression that dieting is the answer to every figure problem. Today, with the advent of scientific weight training, this myth is being rapidly dispelled, but like most myths, it is being dispelled very slowly.

Dieting to lose weight results in the overall reduction of body size rather than in toning and firming specific body parts. A fat woman looks in the mirror and says to herself, "My stomach is popping out, my butt is diving to the pavement, and my thighs look like tree trunks. I have to go on a diet." So she diets very strictly for a month and loses 10 pounds. But when she looks in the mirror she is disappointed. She says to herself, "I still look fat. What's wrong?"

I see it everywhere—at the supermarket, shopping in Beverly Hills, in restaurants—women who are big versions of a fat person and women who are little versions of a fat person, all of them still fat.

Dieting alone can do just so much. It reduces your size and your weight, but it cannot reshape specific parts of your body. Only working with weights the right way can do that. Since fat tends to accumulate more on the buttocks and abdominal areas of a woman, she will see some change in those areas as dieting removes fat from the body. Unfortunately, those areas are still left soft and flabby rather than tight and firm—*unless* she also begins to work out correctly to develop the muscles there.

WHAT ABOUT AEROBICS?

Because aerobic exercise is an effective aid to weight loss and strengthens heart and lungs, I am very much in favor of it. Ideally, I recommend three thirty-minute aerobic sessions per week. Your health will benefit, and you'll find you have more stamina when performing your body shaping exercise routines.

If you are overweight, aerobic exercise can be particularly valuable. The only way to get rid of fat is to burn it off, and aerobic exercise helps you do that more efficiently and faster—and more enjoyably!

All you have to do in aerobic exercise is get your pulse rate up to 70 to 80 percent of maximum capacity and keep it there for at least twenty minutes. (To determine your maximum pulse rate, just subtract your age from 220.) You can accomplish that with any of a number of activities—cycling, jogging or running, walking briskly, aerobic dancing, swimming, even cleaning house energetically. Whatever activity you prefer is fine, as long as you sustain the elevated pulse rate for at least twenty minutes and do it at least three times a week.

Don't try to jump to a full twenty or thirty minutes of aerobics if you're not accustomed to vigorous physical activity. (And confer with your physician before starting a program of aerobics if you've any health condition that may be affected.) Work up to a full aerobic routine slowly. Do three five-minute sessions the first week, three ten-minute sessions for the next two weeks, and increase the time by five additional minutes every two weeks until you reach thirty minutes. If it takes you longer, that's all right, too.

As beneficial as aerobic exercise is, however, it's not enough to reshape your body to the perfect proportions you'd like to see reflected in your mirror. To accomplish that you've got to do more than burn off fat; you've got to build and shape your muscle. It may be satisfying to see fat dropping off your frame, but in the long run, wouldn't you rather build in curves and firm flesh where you want it rather than just settle for a somewhat thinner shapelessness?

WHY THIS PROGRAM WORKS!

There are no gimmicks involved here; *you will see worthwhile results.* I've worked with thousands of women ever since I started working out myself, and I've discovered that scientific weight training *does* work. It changes undesirable, unshapely body parts into perfectly formed, sensual body parts.

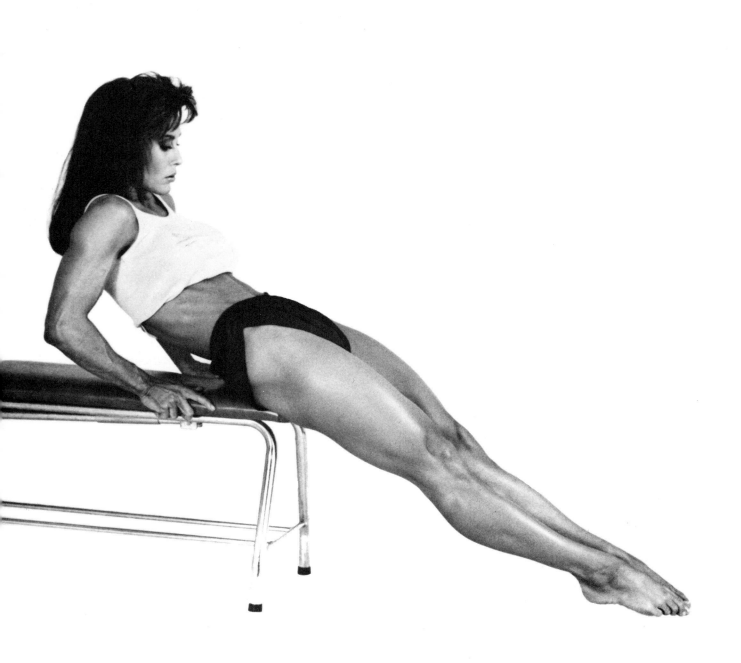

The program in this book is the result of years of experimentation. Each exercise has been carefully selected to challenge each muscle or muscle group at just the right angle and thereby create a perfect body formed of perfect parts.

5

WILL IT TAKE LONG TO SEE RESULTS?

The good news is clear—you can in effect spot reduce by spot building. But how long will that take?

Provided you conscientiously follow the routine(s) given in this book for the part(s) you are focusing on, you'll experience a sense of change within a matter of weeks. You'll feel the muscle(s) growing stronger; depending on the body part, your general physical condition, your genetic heritage, and to some extent your age, you'll start to see the reshaping process begin.

If you are very overweight, the reshaping effects may not be immediately apparent. Even though your muscles are developing tone and increasing in size, they may remain hidden under a layer of fat. For example, if you are more than 10 pounds overweight, you will not easily see the development of your abdominal muscles; if you are more than 15 pounds overweight, you will not easily see the progress you are making in the buttock and thigh areas. Development will be more readily evident in other parts of your body, because they do not tend to accumulate fat to the extent that the abdominal, buttock, and thigh areas do.

WELCOME TO THE CLUB

You're tired of feeling dissatisfied with your body. You're fed up with programs that promise you the world and then give you nothing for your precious time and your hard-earned money. You've come to realize that if you want to get results you should go to an expert—someone who demonstrates in her own life the effectiveness of what she teaches. You're ready to work smart. Welcome to the club. In a short time you will see a complete transformation of the body part(s) you now hate. If you follow the program prescribed in this book, you'll join the growing number of women who have taken control of their bodies and their lives. We're happy to have you in the club.

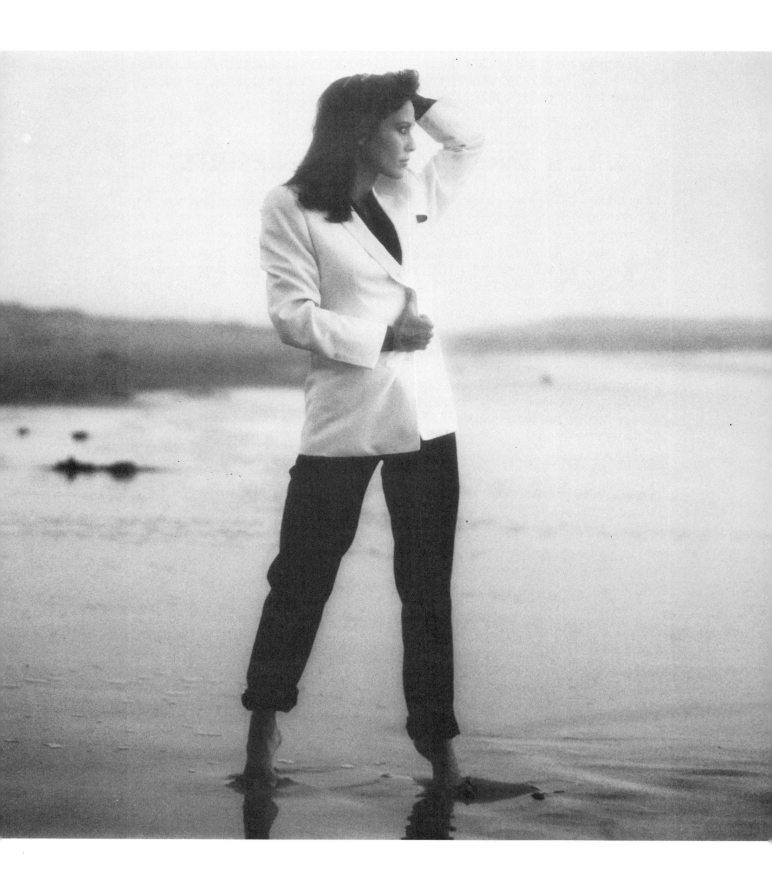

2

How Long Will It Take to See Results?

Results depend upon a lot of things: your present condition, your genetic composition, your age, your previous involvement in physical activities, your diet, your metabolism, your enthusiasm, and most important, *your commitment*.

However, *everyone* who follows this program will see results. The time range for achieving a transformed body part varies from one to six months, but everyone will see some improvement between two weeks and two months. Let's break it down so you won't be disappointed if you are not one of the lucky ones who will see results in two weeks.

Be aware that even within the following groups, there is room for variation. Each person reading this book is in a different stage in life. Each of you brings to this program a given mental set. For this reason, although we may tell you, "If you are between twenty and thirty-three you should see results in this amount of time," you may see results twice as fast because *your* body may respond to the weights more quickly and because you are especially highly motivated.

No matter what your mind-set, genetic composition, or exercise history, you can be sure of this: You will see results in time.

Here's an approximate time-scale for you. Read through your "category," but don't limit yourself to it. Use it as a guideline only.*

*These guidelines are based on a four-year study of women in South Texas from 1977 to 1981 at Sport Palace Association in Harlingen, Texas. Documented results are kept on file.

8 ░ ACTIVE MOST OF YOUR LIFE AND BETWEEN THE AGES OF TWENTY AND THIRTY-THREE

You have always been active. You used to walk a lot, you were involved in various sports in your high school days, and you have continued to participate in various physical activities. You are still active and yet you notice that things are beginning to "go." You look in the mirror and you wonder, "Is this cellulite forming?" or you say, "My body seems to be getting loose." You are genetically gifted, so you're a bit shocked to see your body losing its tone. You never seemed to have to work at keeping in shape before. Now you're getting scared—at times even desperate.

Do not despair. You can see results as early as two weeks. Of course, where you see results will depend upon your genetic composition, which is different from that of other women. Since most women share the problem areas that take extra time, we'd venture a guess that it won't be your buttocks or abdominal area that will show results first. However, you may see a tightening up in your upper body—your chest, shoulders, and back. Your arms will feel stronger and you may perceive a firm muscle forming in your biceps area. Your triceps may take a little longer.

In two months your entire body will experience an uplifted look (assuming, of course, that you are working your entire body). At this point your legs will show development and your buttocks and abdominal area will begin to look a lot tighter and feel a lot firmer.

In two to three months your body parts will obviously be taking on a new shape. People will begin to comment. "What have you been doing?" they'll ask, knowing that it obviously isn't just another diet. In six months you will have a perfectly formed body part or body, depending upon whether or not you've chosen to work your entire body. If you've worked your entire body, you may find yourself proud to display the results in a bikini. You'll be close to perfect—or perfect for you.

FAIRLY ACTIVE MOST OF YOUR LIFE AND BETWEEN THE AGES OF THIRTY-FOUR AND FORTY-FIVE

You will see results, but it will take you a little longer. For example, a forty-year-old may have to wait three to four weeks before seeing any visible results and experiencing an overall tightening. You may have to wait four months to see a total uplifting of the body and six months to see major changes—that is, changes people will notice immediately—and a year to have a body that looks great in a bikini and is nearly perfectly formed.

YOU'VE NEVER DONE A HARD DAY'S EXERCISE IN YOUR LIFE—A "SKINNY FAT" BETWEEN TWENTY AND THIRTY-THREE

9

You've always looked good in clothing because you're slim. You even used to look pretty good in a bathing suit, at least when you were a teenager—or you thought so at the time. Now you see your body in the nude and you don't like what you see. When you take off your clothes you're ashamed of yourself, and you don't like the feeling.

In one month you'll feel a lot better. You won't see much in the way of visible results, but you'll feel so good that you'll think you look better. In fact, sometimes when you look in the mirror you'll swear you see changes, then at other times you'll see nothing and feel disappointed, even confused.

If you're in this group, you have a lot of body fat clinging to your body, even though you are not overweight. It takes time to remove this body fat and replace it with firm muscle. But you will do it—in time.

In three months you'll see some definite changes. You'll be generally tighter, and your posture will improve. Your arms will show shape and some definition, and when you press your finger into your thigh, it will no longer sink in and almost get lost in the "mush." Instead it will bounce back because your thighs will have become toned. The same will be true for every other part of your body.

In six months everyone will comment on your changing body, and in a year you will be proud of yourself in the nude. You'll be amazed that you could have achieved such a body. You'll say to yourself, "And all this time I thought I had poor genetics." It may have taken you a little longer than someone who is genetically gifted, but who cares? What's the big deal if it takes you six months to a year instead of three months to six months? Once you get there, it's yours! You have it for life as long as you keep exercising regularly, and by then you'll enjoy it so much you won't want to ever give it up.

YOU'VE NEVER DONE A HARD DAY'S EXERCISE IN YOUR LIFE—A "SKINNY FAT" BETWEEN THIRTY-FOUR AND FORTY-FIVE

You will feel better after the first workout, if aches and pains from muscles that haven't been worked before constitute feeling better (we think so). But it will be about three weeks before you start to feel generally more fit. It will take about six weeks to two months before you really feel great. Think of it as acquiring a taste for excellence.

In two months you'll see a hint of change here, a shadow of development there. In four months you'll see definite development of certain body parts. Your shoulders will begin to show more muscular shape, your thighs will become a bit tighter, your buttocks will seem to be lifting and your abdominal area will show some improvement.

In six months you'll see a lot more. Some of your body parts will command complimentary attention from friends.

It will take you about a year to have a dramatically improved body, and maybe a bit longer to achieve a perfect body. But who cares? Working out is a process. It's a continual "improving" and growing and developing. Instead of atrophying and wilting, your body will be tightening and taking on a more pleasing shape. Instead of feeling older, your body will literally feel and look younger. Time is going to happen anyway. You might as well do something wonderful in it.

YOU ARE FAT OR OBESE, 15 TO 50 POUNDS OVERWEIGHT, AND BETWEEN TWENTY AND FORTY-FIVE

Change begins immediately, but you will not see visible results for a while, as they occur on a microscopic level. Your muscles will develop slowly, at first still under the layers of fat. As you continue to work out *and* eat properly (see Perfect Diet, Chapter 16), your fat will gradually diminish and your newly shaped body will begin to show through.

You will feel stronger and more fit in about a month. In three months you'll notice visible shades of difference. Depending upon how much fat is still covering your body, some muscles will begin to show through. No matter how overweight you were, you will have lost at least 15 pounds of fat by now. Your posture will have improved because of the fat loss and muscular development.

After six months of working out and eating properly, all body parts will show major changes. And in a year, you'll be at your goal or very close to it. Don't think it's an impossible dream. Even if you are 100 pounds overweight, this program will work for you. *You can do it!*

WHAT ABOUT WOMEN OVER FORTY-FIVE?

You can count yourself in on the promised results. It may take you a little longer, but you certainly will see the results. We've seen some ladies in their late forties, early fifties, and even their sixties transform particular body parts—even their entire bodies.

Many women over forty-five choose to work on their triceps. They want to develop this muscle because they don't like the way the flesh in their upper arms sags and waves whenever they raise their arms. The triceps is located between the armpit and the elbow, on the "back"of your arm. As you get older, this area tends to jiggle and look unappealing when you raise your arm, because the natural muscle has gradually shrunken or atrophied a little each year after age thirty.

Women who have followed this program have transformed their sagging triceps into firm, tight muscles. If you are over forty-five, you can still write your own ticket. Don't worry about how long it takes. You might be surprised. One sixty-three-year-old grandmother who followed this program is now striking "triceps poses" when she attends family functions. It took her only four months to achieve this remarkable transformation of her previously sagging triceps.

Don't let your sense of age limit you. Work on your body and expect the best results. Yes, it may take you longer than a younger woman to reach your goal, but you may also surprise yourself—and those around you. Maybe you will put the younger crowd to shame and achieve results in some areas more quickly than they do. Go for it.

THE KEY TO SUCCESS

In order to ensure success with this program, you must make a commitment. If you make the commitment and stick with it, results are as inevitable as the law of gravity. Don't let impatience rob you of the opportunity to have a newly formed body and a new outlook on life. Hang in there. Success is just around the corner.

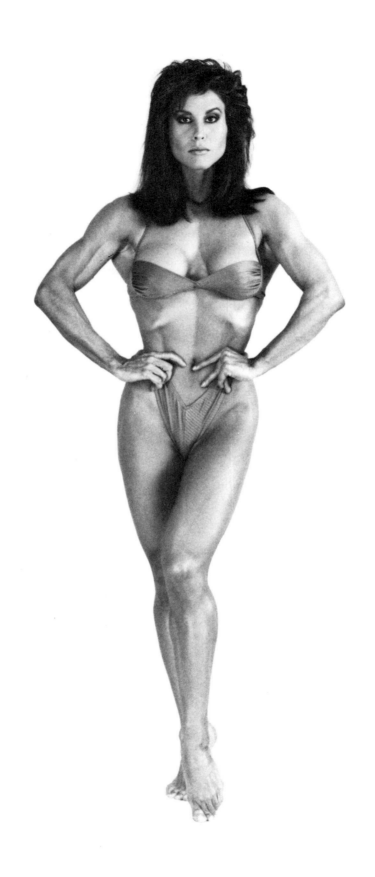

3

Attitude Is Everything

When it comes to working out, attitude is everything. Your attitude is your way of looking at a given situation. What is the situation you're looking at right now, while you're reading this page? It's the situation of your body in the shape it's in now and what you will have to do in order to get it into shape.

Stop right now and think. What is your attitude about this situation? Are you thinking, "I'll probably have to work like a fiend, and it will probably take months before I see results. Oh well, I guess I have no choice. You have to pay the price if you want to look good."

Wrong attitude. When you go to do your exercises, you should think of it as "fun time." Remember when you were a child and you played all day long in the playground? Your mother had a hard time getting you to come home for dinner. You didn't know it then, but you were working out pretty hard—climbing up and down the bars, swinging from one bar to another, pushing up and down on the seesaw, pumping back and forth on the swing. And you had the right attitude about working out. You couldn't wait to get back to that playground again. You looked forward to all that "work," not as work but as play.

Children don't think of activity on playground gyms as work because they let their bodies do what is natural. It is only as we get older and become bogged down by the busy schedule of adult life that we begin to develop the wrong attitude about exercise. We see it as an intrusion in our lives—a burden, more "work" thrust upon us. It requires

13

14

our expending energy, putting out effort, and we resent it. But that's a self-defeating attitude.

The body doesn't lie. Children run and romp and "work out" because their bodies demand it of them. Before our technological society settled us in offices and in front of computer terminals, people got plenty of exercise performing physical tasks, and they enjoyed their work. Work—using the muscles of the body, developing strength and physical prowess—is the most natural thing in the world. It's probably because of our hectic schedules that we've developed stress-related attitudes about engaging in physical activities.

Push aside your present attitudes of dread and distaste for what is coming up—if you dare. Let your real self come through, the you who is excited about stimulating your body, the you who looks forward to "working out" the way you did when you were a child. The child in you is alive and well. That child has been forced into the background, but now it's time to bring that child forth again.

So many people are afraid to be childlike because they confuse it with being "childish." It's okay to be childlike. No one is telling you to become immature. I'm telling you to realize that your body wants to enjoy a carefree workout. In other words, your body wants to be stimulated, to have fun. Why not let it do just that?

It won't take long for you to believe that, because it's true. Exercise *is* fun. People begin a workout with a load of problems and walk away feeling unburdened and uplifted, on a natural high. Why? Because the body experiences a physical euphoria as an increased supply of blood circulates throughout the muscles. When you think of it, a physical high is what people reach for when they do drugs, only that high is unnatural. A workout high is a natural high. The euphoria you experience comes without the price of damage to your body and a hangover the next day. In fact, the opposite occurs. Your body is helped, not damaged, and the next day you feel great instead of miserable. No wonder doctors routinely prescribe exercise for patients who are tense and even neurotic.

YOUR ATTITUDE IN FRONT OF THE MIRROR

When you look in the mirror, what do you see? Do you focus on your "unsatisfactory" body part and tell yourself something like, "Disgusting. It would take a miracle to do anything with this"? As you flip through the pictures here, do you think, "It's easy for Rachel and Joyce to talk, look at their bodies," and then conclude, "there's no hope for me; this will never work"?

Wrong attitude. (You should have seen my thighs and Joyce's butt before we started working out.)

Make up your mind right now to adopt a new attitude toward your "unsatisfactory" body part. Think of it as being in a state of metamorphosis, a state of gradual change. You weren't born with that body part in that condition. Your body grew and changed as you evolved through the various stages of your life. Then when you became an adult, some of your body parts began to lose tone and shape. They changed in a negative direction because of neglect. But now you can begin to affect the direction in which your body—any part you choose to work on—will change. Your body is evolving, but from now on it's going to become more shapely, firm rather than flabby. Instead of losing muscle tone, you will be gaining it.

Your new attitude will be: "I can't wait to see the changes I'm going to make in this body part." Look in the mirror at your previously "undesirable" body part, but now see it as it really is—in a stage of metamorphosis or change, only now *you are in control* of the change. You will control the change by following the workouts prescribed in this book and by using your mind to help you get to your goal.

VISUALIZATION IN FRONT OF THE MIRROR

Stand in front of the mirror, look at your "unsatisfactory" body part, and imagine it being transformed into the perfectly formed body part you've always dreamed of. Where up to now you've focused on flab or unattractive angularity, "see" the muscles underneath. They are there, just waiting for you to awaken them to shapely development. Imagine them responding to the attention you are paying them. Look at the points where you will see lift. Picture the progressive change as the muscle fills out, giving you curves where you've always wanted them. See the potential, and then know that's within your reach.

Direct your mind to direct your body. It's not hocus pocus, just plain fact. Your mind is or should be in full control, watching your previously undesirable body part changing before your very eyes.

You will greatly speed up your progress if you do this whenever you look in the mirror. Stop using that mirror time to put yourself down and make negative predictions about yourself.

If you can't picture what you'd like your body part to look like, go through some magazines for a picture of the corresponding body part on a woman whom you admire. Or get a "before" picture of yourself and draw over that picture and reshape your body. Then stand in front of the mirror and, body part by body part, visualize yourself changing into that new perfect body. Remember that your mind determines what your body will do—in more ways than one.

16
YOUR ATTITUDE DURING YOUR ACTUAL WORKOUT—CONCENTRATION

When I pick up a pair of dumbbells to begin my workout, this is what goes on in my mind: First of all, I'm here for a reason. I'm in the gym (or at home) making an effort to do something about my body, and that fact determines my attitude from the start. My efforts are going to be utilized for maximum results, because results and rewards are a big part of what my life is all about.

I like to get excited about my set. Sometimes my attitude is more aggressive than it is at other times—it depends on what's happening in my life at that particular moment. But regardless of the degree of aggression I feel, I make sure I'm emotionally committed to that set. Maybe I'll decide to go a little heavier that day. If that's the case, I'll become mentally charged and imagine myself building super firm, full, shapely muscles that will win me any competition, by whoever's or whatever's standards.

You should approach the weights in the same manner whenever you are feeling especially motivated. Imagine your body being scrutinized by the most critical judge, and imagine that judge being overwhelmed by the perfect symmetry of your body. Picture yourself walking on the beach this summer or disrobing in front of the man of your dreams. Or picture yourself standing before the most critical judge of all—yourself—when you view your body after a shower or before dressing for bed. No longer will you criticize yourself. Instead you'll be delighted at your progress toward perfection.

When in a more delicate mood, I'll approach my set with a different attitude. I see myself sculpting my muscles artistically, much as an artist works to create a masterpiece. I go through the movements with a sense of artistic grace so that the flow of the exercise almost seems like a dance, enjoying and savoring the sensation it brings to my muscles.

The shades of mood in your attitude toward working out will vary, but the commitment will always be the same. You will expect and visualize specific results, and you'll give whatever energy you have to your set. Your reward will be immediate because, as you work out, you'll begin to feel revitalized. During your workout your mood will change from low to high or from high to higher, while your body changes gradually from bad to great or from great to greater.

Now, don't misunderstand. You're under no obligation to leap up and down with joy as you reach for those dumbbells or that barbell. All you have to do is focus your mind on the muscle you are working out and keep your mind concentrated on that muscle throughout your routine. Tell that muscle to grow. Squeeze (flex) it and stretch it, as the instructions indicate. That's the right gym attitude. Concentration.

It is only when you concentrate totally on one thing that your mind is forced to stop concentrating on something else. If you concentrate totally on the muscle you are working out, how can you continue to worry about the argument you had with your boss or the difficulty you're having with your husband or friend? You can't. When you truly concentrate on reshaping—rebuilding—yourself, you forget troubles. Then when you're finished working out, you experience a strange kind of relief. It seems to you as if a burden has been lifted—as if a therapy session has taken place. You have cleared the slate of your mind and you are now free to do some fresh, new thinking.

If you adopt the right attitude when you work out, you'll experience a double benefit. Not only will you give your mind a rest but your muscles will develop at a much faster rate—as much as twice as fast as if you try working out with something else on your mind at the same time.

17

It won't be hard for you to concentrate on an exercise movement if you follow instructions exactly, because doing so will keep your mind focused every second on the muscle you are working. Just flow with the workout for that body part and you'll find yourself concentrating fully—and it will be fun.

Remember these three positives when it comes to working out, and you'll have a wonderful time.

1. *Exercise is fun.* It's a kind of therapy, a minivacation from stress.
2. *Your body is in a state of positive metamorphosis.* See it that way in the mirror.
3. *By focusing your mind on your muscle, you prime it for perfect development.* Approach your set with a definite goal. Give your muscle your full attention. Allow your mood to mold your set, building aggressively or sculpting artistically, depending on how you feel.

EFFECTS IN OTHER AREAS OF YOUR LIFE

Attitude and discipline in your workout will carry over to other areas of your life. You'll find, perhaps to your surprise, that you are generally more in control of things. For example, you may have had trouble cleaning up after a meal, even though you hate to see a messy kitchen. But once you begin working out you may find yourself saying, "I'll do the dishes now. It will only take a few minutes; then I'll feel good for hours when I see the neat, clean kitchen." Or you may see a carry-over in your job situation. Suppose you are considering taking on a long-term project, one that previously you would have had no patience to begin because of your feeling that it would "take forever." But once you've seen the result of your weekly efforts in working out—seen the fruits of steady input (your reshaped body)—you may find it easier to see the long-term results of other tasks and be willing to put in the daily effort required to see them through.

THE THREE BIGGEST MISCONCEPTIONS REGARDING WORKING OUT

Before you begin your workout, we want to be sure that you're not one of the many women who are laboring under three misconceptions we commonly encounter. If you are, rid yourself of these misconceptions now so that your attitude toward working out will be correct.

Misconception #1: I can get in shape by doing aerobics.
As we've already noted, aerobics are excellent for conditioning the heart and lungs.

18

They are effective in burning excess fat from all over your body, but there is no way you can reshape your body by doing aerobic exercises.

In order to reshape your body, you have to work specifically on each targeted body part with *anaerobic* exercises such as the weight-training routines described in this book.

An anaerobic exercise is a high intensity exercise in which an oxygen debt is created and glycogen stored in the muscle being worked is depleted. When you do an anaerobic exercise, your body burns mainly glycogen, which is produced by the carbohydrates you consume. You could not do anaerobics for a half hour without at least fifteen- to thirty-second rests between sets, because your body would run out of energy. You can do aerobic exercises for thirty minutes without resting, however, because they are low intensity and there is an abundant supply of oxygen. Instead of burning a great deal of glycogen, aerobic exercises burn fat. They are not capable, however, of reshaping the body. Only intelligent weight training can do that. I do recommend aerobics as a part of your overall exercise regime to help you gain stamina and burn excess body fat.

Misconception #2: Once I start exercising I have to keep working out until the day I die or else my body will turn to a mound of flab.

You can get over your fear of that right now. Your body *won't* turn into a mound of fat. What *will* happen if you decide to stop working out is that your muscles will gradually shrink back to the size they were before you started working out. They won't turn into fat. The change happens on a microscopic level. Just as it took months for the full transformation from flab to firm, toned muscle, it will take months to lose all the firmness and tone. You will definitely not have more flab than you did before you started simply because you stopped working out.

It will take you at least as long to get "out of shape" as it did to get into shape. For example, if it took you a year to develop perfectly formed buttocks, hips, and thighs, it would take at least a year of not working out before they returned to the condition they were in before you started. They would look no worse than before—unless, of course, you began eating excessively and put so much extra fat on your body that you could not help but look worse. That's another story, and one has nothing to do with the other.

Muscle is muscle and fat is fat. Muscle merely shrinks to what it was before once it is not being challenged to work any longer. Fat will accumulate on a previously trim area if you begin eating more than you burn off on a daily basis.

And listen to this! There is a bonus for you just for having worked out at all. If you stop working out, say for a year, and then you start again, it will take you *half* the time to get into the shape you were in before. For example, say you worked your buttock-abdominal-hip areas for a year and then stopped for a year. You would seem to be back to square one, with those body parts looking like they did before you ever worked out. But underneath, the muscles would be on alert, ready to get tight again. After a relatively short period of working out, they would spring back to the shape you were in after a year of working out. We like to think of this fortunate muscle memory trait as "muscles in the bank."

Give up your unreasoned fear of exercise once and for all. Stop thinking in terms of bondage—"Oh no, I'll have to do this for the rest of my life." You won't have to. But we're betting you'll want to. Anyway, you have nothing to lose by starting—nothing except some flabby muscles and out-of-shape body parts.

Misconception #3: If my clothes start getting tighter, that means I am getting too muscular.

If your pant legs get tighter after working out for a month or two, you should thank God rather than panic. You're lucky—one of those genetically gifted people who respond rapidly to weight training. What is happening is that your muscle is developing a little faster than the fat is melting away. Continue to diet and exercise, and soon the extra fat will be gone and you will have a perfectly formed muscle. Your pant legs may not be any more tight over the long run, but if they are you won't care because in the nude, in the mirror, you will see the most perfectly formed legs you could ever have imagined. So don't panic as soon as you see a muscle developing. That's what it's all about. How do you expect to reshape your body without building up muscles? Muscles are what give shape to your body. You have to have something to put on your bones. Is it going to be soft, flabby fat or firm, shapely muscles? The decision is yours.

There are probably fifty other fears based on misconceptions, but I don't want to run through all of them. They don't concern me. "Will I get hurt?" "Will men like my body?" "What about the women who use steroids?"

You won't get hurt if you follow the instructions in this book. Yes, virtually any man will like your body better when it is firm and toned. (But we're not miracle workers either. We can't guarantee that now you will automatically have every man in town after you. But it may happen, so watch out.) And forget about steroids. They are taken by only a few women involved in bodybuilding, powerlifting, and other competitive sports. These artificial male hormones give them strength and size, but these advantages go paired with side effects that lead to a loss of natural femininity, not to mention health hazards and possible death.

THE CONCLUSION OF
THE WHOLE MATTER

Adjust your attitude now. If you have been imagining all the drawbacks associated with working out, start thinking about all the positive benefits. Erase the past. If you have allowed yourself to become discouraged as a result of past attempts at getting into shape—attempts that failed—clear your mind and record a new message: "The reason my past attempts failed is clear. I did not work intelligently or consistently [whatever the case may be]. With this carefully designed body parts shaping program, I *will* transform my body into its most perfect form. It *will* work. The results are inevitable if I follow the program."

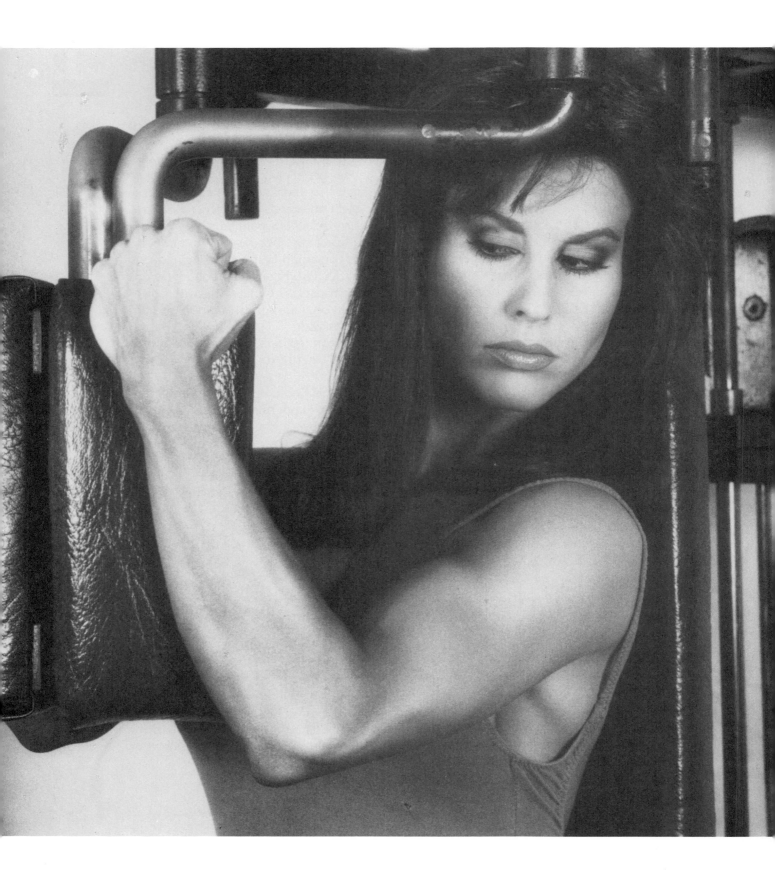

4

Body Shaping Basics

To begin with, every specialized activity has its own special language, and this is no exception. So before you start, you'll want to familiarize yourself with the terms used to describe equipment you will be using and aspects of the exercise routines themselves.

Let's start with the equipment.

WORKOUT EQUIPMENT

Free weights. Barbells and dumbbells. They are called "free weights" because they are not permanently attached to the floor, as are machines, and can be carried around the gym or home exercise area at will.

Barbell. A metal bar that holds various weighted plates at either end and is designed to be held and balanced with both hands. Some barbells have permanently attached weights; others can be disassembled to change the weights as desired, with the weight held in place by a collar.

Dumbbell. A short metal bar with either a permanently fixed weight on either end or changeable plates held in place with a collar. It is designed to be held in one hand.

22

Collar. A holding device placed on either end of a barbell or dumbbell after the weighted plates have been added so that these do not shift or fall off the bar.

Plates. Disc-shaped weights that can be added to either end of a barbell or dumbbell. They vary in size. A typical weight progression is 2½ pounds, 5 pounds, 10 pounds, 25 pounds, 45 pounds. Plates are also available in kilogram increments.

Machines. Any of a variety of devices specially designed to exercise one or other body part, often operated with the use of pulleys or cams to control the weight resistance that is applied. Because of the greater element of control, machines are generally considered safer than free weights. Depending on the machine and the exercise being performed, they may also be more effective than free weights. They are necessary to provide variety in the workout, and some machines—the lat pull-down machine, the pec deck machine, the cable crossover machine, etc.—are virtually indispensable, although there are free weight substitutes for most exercises performed on a machine (and vice versa). Bally Life Circuit, Cybex, Eagle, Nautilus, Universal, Paramount, and Kaiser are some of the more popular brand-name machines.

Flat exercise bench. A long, narrow, padded bench of standard height and parallel to the floor, specifically designed for exercise purposes. Flat bench flyes, seated side laterals, and cross-face triceps extensions are examples of exercises done on the flat exercise bench.

Incline exercise bench. An exercise bench that can be raised to a 45-degree incline. Incline bench presses and incline flyes are two examples of exercises performed on the incline bench. Since an incline bench can also be placed in a flat position, you can also use it for any exercise done on a flat exercise bench and thus save yourself the purchase price of a separate flat bench.

Decline exercise bench. A bench that is on a decline of up to 45 degrees, with roller pads or some other holding device for the feet, used for exercises such as the decline dumbbell press and sit-ups.

EXERCISE TERMINOLOGY

Exercise. The specific movement you perform in order to strengthen and develop a muscle or muscle group—for example, a sit-up, leg press, incline flye, calf raise, or side lateral.

Repetition, or rep. One complete movement of any exercise from start to finish. At completion of a repetition you will be in the start position again.

Set. A number of repetitions performed in sequence without pausing for a rest between reps.

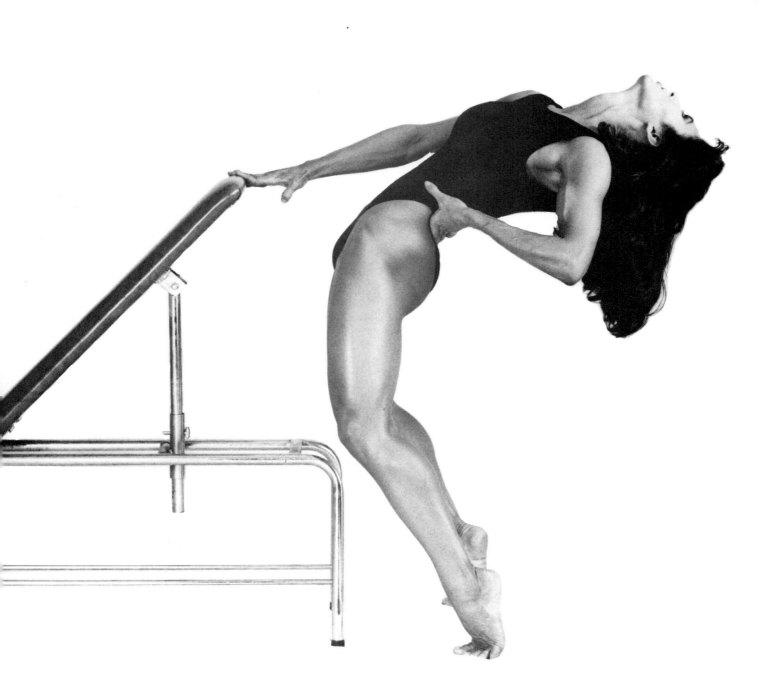

24

Rest. The brief pause between sets (it's usually about thirty seconds but may be as much as sixty seconds) to allow your muscle(s) to recover enough strength to perform the next set.

Routine. The combination of exercises performed in a given sequence for a particular body part.

Resistance. The amount of weight used in an exercise to stress the muscles sufficiently to stimulate development.

Muscle isolation. The process of working a body part independently of other body parts. Because of difference in structure, function, and work capacity, you ensure maximum development of a particular muscle or muscle group through exercise routines that focus stress entirely or primarily on that muscle.

Stress. The intense physical challenge provided by an exercise to stimulate muscle development/growth.

Weight progression. The gradual, progressive addition of weight resistance to a workout routine as weights used in exercises become so easy to lift that there is no longer sufficient stress on the target muscle(s) to stimulate further development/growth. Because weight progression is a clear indication of increased muscle capabilities, it is a natural measure of progress. (It doesn't matter how quickly you progress. As long as you work hard and do make progress, you'll find your muscles gradually taking on the tone, shape, and proportion you're aiming for.)

MUSCLE GROWTH AND SHAPE

After you've been working out for a while (at least a month), you will begin to see changes in some of your working muscles. The terms given here describe what you are affecting or will see happen.

Definition. Muscularity that is relatively free of surrounding fat. The combination of muscle development and absence or elimination of fat leads to a clearly visible, or defined, outline of muscle shape.

Density. The quality of hardness in a muscle. A dense muscle is well formed, well defined, and very hard.

Pumped up. The temporary enlargement of muscle tissue due to increased blood flow to the muscle as a result of strenuous exercise. After a few minutes, but sometimes an hour or more, the muscle returns to normal size. Seeing a "pump" in your muscle is cause for satisfaction. It means the muscle is responding to the stimulus you've provided to make it grow.

WORKING OUT AT HOME

Whether you work out at home or in a fitness center will depend on your schedule, your preferences, and/or your finances. There are definite advantages to working out at home (as there are advantages to working out in a health club gym).

Working out at home saves you the time of travel to the gym. This is especially a factor if you are focusing on only one or two body parts. Since you may be spending only fifteen to thirty minutes two or three times a week to go through your routines, why spend double or triple the amount of time to get to and from a health club, particularly when you can work out effectively at home?

Furthermore, if you work out at home, you can do so at any time of day—or night. You're not limited to health club hours. What's more, you never have to wait for the equipment to be available. You have exclusive rights.

You also have complete privacy. You don't have to suffer the embarrassment of people watching you struggle as a beginner (although it won't be long before you'll be expert in performing your exercise movements).

You save money. You make a small initial investment in some home equipment and then you have it for life. There's no yearly health club membership fee. If you stop working out for a while, whatever the reason, you don't lose money. As you might guess, most gyms will not extend the membership period for members who stop working out for weeks or months at a time. At home you can go back to working out whenever you like; the equipment is always there.

When working out at home it's easy to break up your workout. For example, if you are doing only your buttocks and abdominals, you can do the routine for one in the morning and the other in the evening. If you work out at a gym, you certainly won't want to travel back and forth twice a day for two fifteen-minute workouts.

PURCHASING HOME GYM EQUIPMENT

What you purchase naturally depends on which body part(s) you decide to focus on.

Here's a summary of what you'll need for each body part. Obviously, if you will be exercising more than one body part, there's no need to duplicate pieces. Query your local equipment supplier on the best combinations for your purposes.

Chest

- A combination incline-decline-flat exercise bench. Look for a multi-purpose model rather than buy three separate pieces.
- Set of dumbbells, with variable weights to allow for a total of 10, 15, 20, and 25 pounds for either dumbbell
- Standard barbell set, with a 25-pound stripped bar and changeable plates of 2½, 5, and 10 pounds weight

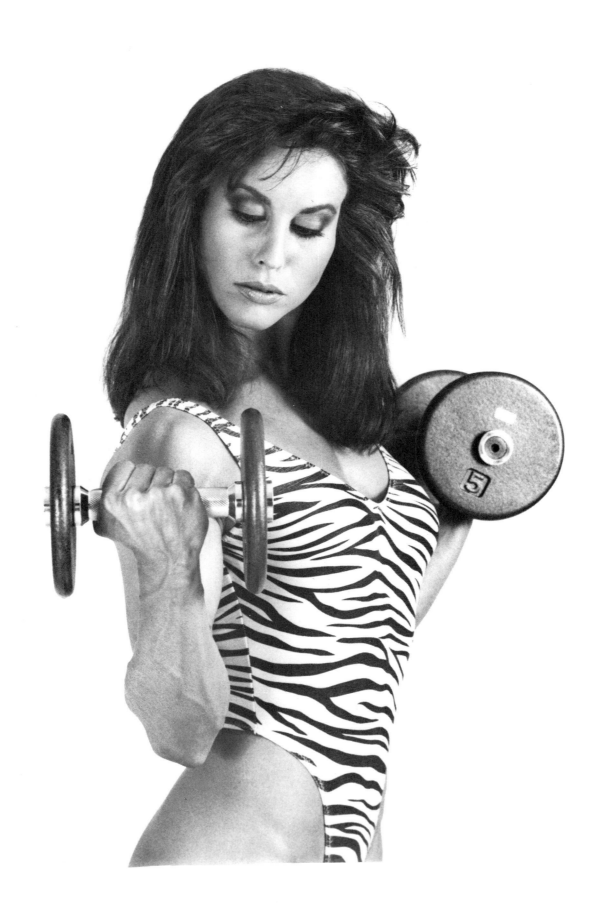

Shoulders

- Set of dumbbells, with variable weights to build to totals of 5, 8, 10, 12, and 15 pounds for either dumbbell
- Standard barbell set, with 25-pound stripped bar and changeable plates of 2½, 5, and 10 pounds weight

Back

- Set of dumbbells, with variable weights to build to a total of 5, 10, 15, 20, and 25 pounds for either dumbbell (possibly more, depending on your strength and state of development)

Biceps

- Set of dumbbells, with variable weights to build to a total of 10, 12, 15, and 20 pounds for either dumbbell

Triceps

- Set of dumbbells, with variable weights to build to totals of 5, 8, 10, 12, 15, and 20 pounds for either dumbbell

Abdominals

- Incline-decline-flat exercise bench. Look for a combination model.

Buttocks

- Ankle weights with slots for additional weights plus weights of 1 pound and 3 pounds (in sets). However, you can also simply use a pair of heavy shoes initially.

Thighs

- One dumbbell, with variable weights to build to a total of 5, 10, 15, and 20 pounds
- Standard barbell set, with 25-pound stripped bar and sets of plates weighing 2½, 5, 10, and 25 pounds for addition

28 Calves

- A six-inch high wooden platform. (You can also use the edge of a step, if this is conveniently placed.)
- One dumbbell, with variable weights to build to a total of 20, 25, and 30 pounds

As your muscles begin to grow and become stronger, you may find that you have to buy a few more plates to add to your barbell or dumbbell set. It may take you anywhere from three weeks to three months to reach that point. Don't rush it. Let it happen naturally.

WORKING OUT AT A FITNESS CENTER OR HEALTH CLUB

The main advantage to belonging to a fitness center or health club is the generally superior quality and greater variety of equipment available to you. But there are other significant advantages as well.

The most notable of these is probably the atmosphere or ambience. The minute you walk through the door your mind automatically turns to your workout. That's what being there is all about; that's what everyone else there has come to do. You can feel the energy around you—positive energy focused on getting and keeping fit and in shape.

I've got a laugh from thousands of women I've spoken to with this comment, but it's absolutely true: "The most difficult exercise you will ever encounter—and one that will stand in the way of your progress many times—is *getting to the gym*." You can always think of something else to be doing. But once you're there, there's an immediate "rush"; you can hardly wait to get into your workout clothes and really make it happen. And you aren't subject to the kind of interruptions you have to deal with at home—ringing telephones, people coming to the door, distractions from family members.

Of course, the quality of the facilities and the service offered makes a considerable difference. Fortunately, fitness centers have come a long way since the advent of the fitness "craze" several years ago. At one time there were health clubs, gyms, fitness centers for women, etc., sprouting up everywhere, and not all of these were conscientiously run or maintained. The objective often seemed to be simply to sell as many memberships as possible, with promises that were never fulfilled and at times with facilities closing within weeks or a few months of soliciting memberships. These circumstances were reflected in comments I made in my first book, *Flex Appeal by Rachel*:

Physical fitness has become a very big industry, with Americans spending billions of dollars each year on gadgets, clothing, spa dues, and special foods. But many people are being ripped off. Besides receiving subpar instruction in aerobics classes, people often waste their time on resistance training, because the instructors simply aren't qualified to teach it. . . . I feel that gym owners and instructors have a responsibility to their members. I don't feel that the average American has to have a degree in exercise physiology just because he or she wants to get in shape. You should be educated by the gym instructors (who should be educated), who have been letting women down for years.

I'm glad to report that the fitness industry has evolved to the point where it's easier to find well-equipped facilities under reputable management almost anywhere in the country. But that doesn't mean you shouldn't shop carefully for a center that suits your needs best.

When choosing a gym or fitness center, it's a good idea to pick one that's fairly close to either home or work. You won't want to spend a lot of time traveling back and forth. That makes it too easy to skip workouts when you've got a busy schedule. And anyway, who has that much time to waste?

You also want a facility where you feel welcome and comfortable. First impressions are very important. The manner in which you're greeted on your first visit is often a good indication of the reception you can expect each time you walk through the door.

You may or may not feel comfortable working out at a gym or fitness center where other people appear more interested in socializing than exercising. What other people do doesn't have to affect you, of course, but you may prefer to avoid a situation where you are tempted into wasting precious workout time.

The quality of instruction or training assistance is particularly important. It would bother me to see instructors giving unequal time to different members. You and the little old lady in baggy leotards deserve every bit as much attention and genuine encouragement as the next person. Also, there's a fine line between supervised instruction and hawk-eyed inspection of your every move. You deserve and should have complete freedom to do whatever exercises you decide on in whatever order you prefer. (Naturally, you should follow proper gym etiquette and observe common courtesy.)

You should be allowed to take this or any other exercise book to the gym without the gym owner or instructor frowning at you. Nowadays there are so many "personal trainers" and self-declared fitness experts that it's not uncommon to find yourself in a situation where the gym management insists on dictating exactly what routines members should follow. Discuss your expectations with the gym or club management. Make it clear that you want the flexibility of following your own judgment but also want someone available to assist you with an exercise if that is necessary.

It's absolutely essential that the facility should be clean and orderly throughout. Besides that, make sure the available equipment includes all the basics necessary for the workouts given in this book. Virtually every gym you might investigate will have what's needed, as I've stuck to basics in setting out the routines here. You may still want to see what else is available, or even reassure yourself that there is enough equipment so that you are not forever competing with others for its use. Anything extra is a bonus—it's always worthwhile trying out new apparatus. You'll find that some are excellent for your purposes, while others are perhaps not suited to your needs.

30

WHAT SHOULD YOU FEEL?

No doubt you've heard the expression "No pain, no gain." That may have led you to expect that you have to torture your muscles to stimulate them to growth. Well, that's not so, but you will probably experience some muscle soreness or ache after a routine of movements that work your muscles to the point of failure—that is, to the point where another movement is impossible without an intervening rest.

So what can you expect, and how can you tell the difference between normal soreness and a pain that signals injury?

I've heard women who began on this kind of exercise program for the first time say things like "I can't move!" or "I think I need a wheelchair" after a vigorous workout. Some will even report the next day that "It was hard getting out of bed" or say, "Hold on, I'll need a minute to negotiate the stairs." But they'll have a mysterious smile on their face, reflecting that somehow they also feel an awakening inner vitality. They've realized and accepted that the soreness they feel is a normal muscle response to stimulation after months or years of neglect. And even that's largely avoidable. If you use the easy break-in system described in the next chapter, any soreness you feel will be easily bearable.

Soreness comes from microscopic tears in the connective tissues (ligaments and tendons) and from the minimal, invisible internal swelling that accompanies those tears. It is the internal swelling in particular that causes the discomfort. This swelling is caused by fluid that immediately surrounds the tear to protect and help repair the tissue there.

It sounds more awful than it is. This kind of tearing happens every time we work a little harder than usual, whether exercising or working around the house. In fact, it's the signal to the body that it must grow stronger, develop more muscle in order to keep up with the demands being made on it. Ordinary muscle soreness is nothing to worry about.

The worst thing you can do in response to muscle soreness is stop working out until it completely goes away. If you do that, you will only get sore again the next time you work out. You must work out the next workout day, even if it is uncomfortable at first. *Be sure to warm up thoroughly first.* Then by the time you finish your routine, the stiff, sore body part will have been massaged by the repetitions of the workout. Blood will have circulated through the sore muscle, making it feel revitalized and less sore.

If you have been a little overenthusiastic in your initial workout or two, the best medicine for the soreness that results is a long, hot bath. Cycling or another low intensity aerobic workout will also help flush out cellular wastes that may have built up and contribute to muscle soreness.

After two to three weeks of regular workouts you should find that soreness has become pretty much a thing of the past. However, if you work out for a few months, stop for a few weeks, and then return to working out, you will feel sore again for a few days. Unless muscle is stimulated regularly it gets lazy, and its first response to restimulation is soreness. There's no reason at all to be concerned. It's simply part of waking your muscles up to regular activity.

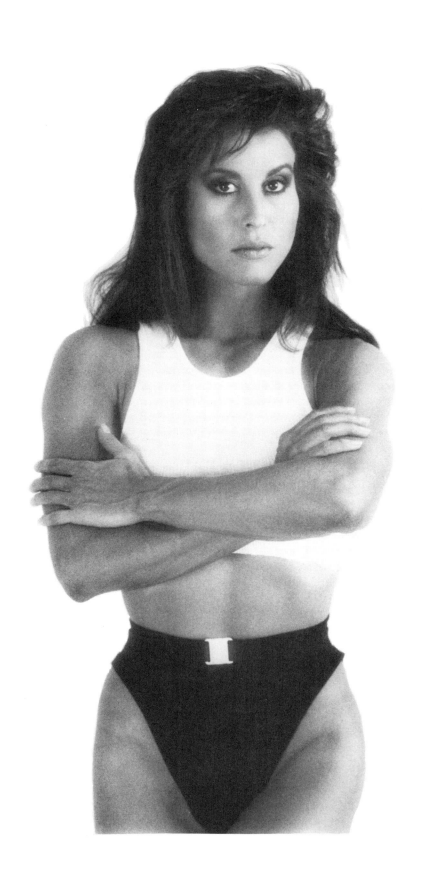

32

HOW DO YOU KNOW IF YOU'RE INJURED?

If some muscle soreness is normal, then how do you recognize a sign of injury?

Injury produces *sharp or incapacitating* pain. You know right away that something is wrong.

To avoid injury, be sure you follow all exercise instructions carefully. Concentrate on proper form and maintaining continuous tension. Don't lift weights that are too heavy for you; never jerk or throw the weights. And always take time to warm up properly.

Most injuries occur because of carelessness. Fascia injuries (those that tear the fascia, or covering of the muscle) happen when you jerk or pull a weight in an abrupt manner. If such an injury occurs, you'll experience deep pain and visible swelling. You'll have to use cold packs to contain the swelling and consult your doctor for further treatment.

Jerking or pulling a weight in an abrupt manner can also lead to stretching or tearing a ligament. If this happens, you will immediately feel sharp, nearly unbearable pain. You'll have to apply cold packs, see your doctor for treatment, and rest the area for a few weeks or longer.

Tendonitis, inflammation of a tendon, can result if you try lifting heavy weights without first warming up properly. When it does occur, you'll experience a continual, nagging pain in the area. The best thing to do then is consult your doctor for treatment.

So long as you follow the warm-up instructions given in this book, you're not likely to experience an injury problem. Unlike sports in which the play of a ball or an opponent controls your actions, working out with weights is a matter of your totally controlling every movement. When you are doing a barbell curl, no one is throwing the barbell at you; you are lifting it alone. No one is telling you to use a weight that is too heavy for you; the decision on what weight to use is yours. You determine what challenge your biceps or other muscles are ready for. Listen to your body, and whatever technique or routine you use to maximize the effectiveness of your training, follow the instructions carefully.

WORKING AROUND INJURY

If you do suffer an injury, however that comes about—perhaps you hurt your elbow playing tennis, or you twisted your ankle walking down the stairs—there's no reason to stop working out completely. See your doctor or physical therapist about the injured part *and continue to work the uninjured body parts.* Ask your doctor if and when you can work the injured part with light weights, or even with no weights at all. Many times a doctor will prescribe just such a workout, as it's been determined that allowing stagnation is the least advisable treatment alternative.

Should your injury require complete rest of that body part for a given time, why not take the opportunity to begin working another body part, one you've previously neglected? This will provide a mental lift in more ways than one. Your positive attitude cannot help but encourage your injury to heal more quickly.

TRAINING PARTNERS

Some people find it's easier to stay motivated and work through a training routine in partnership with another person. You do an exercise set, then your partner does a set, and so on. As long as you don't waste time in conversation during or between sets, this can provide a good pace for many exercises. Furthermore, having a training partner makes it easier to try some intensification techniques, such as forced reps—when you're ready for them. Obviously, the person you work out with regularly has to be someone with a compatible schedule and a compatible personality.

Although competition bodybuilders always work out with a training partner—their high intensity methods require having someone to lend assistance—you won't necessarily need one. If there's someone available who you know would provide helpful support and encouragement, try working out together and see how it goes. But the beauty of the *Perfect Parts* workout is that you can manage it on your own with equally impressive results. *You have what it takes.* You don't need someone else to do it with you or for you.

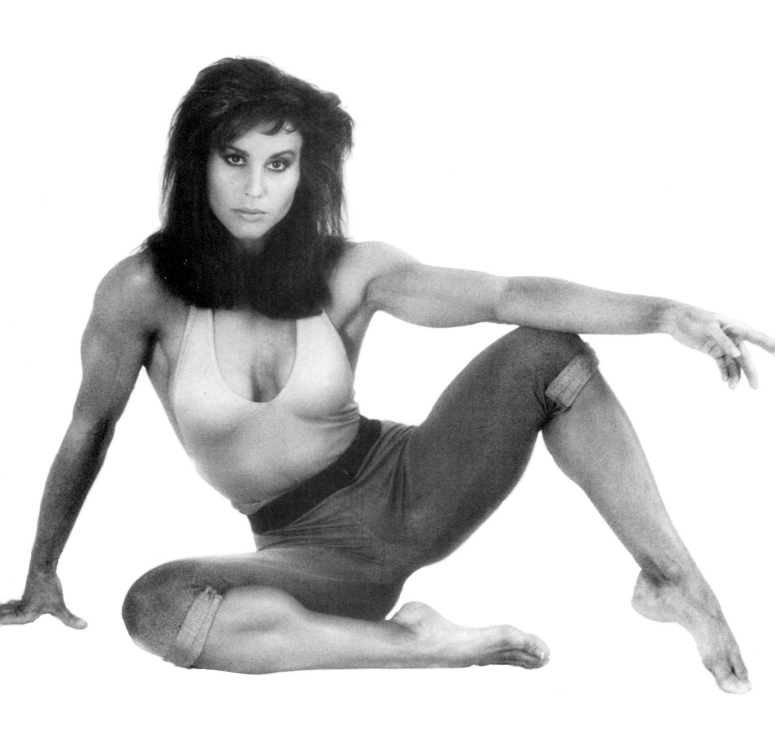

5

How to Use the <u>Perfect Parts</u> Workout

You can do anything you want with this program. You can reshape only one body part, two body parts, three body parts, or every part of your body. It's totally up to you. Of course, I hope you eventually decide to work on your entire body—it will only take an hour of your time three or four days a week to build a totally new you. That's not a bad time investment.

But if you're only interested in working on one or two body parts, that's fine, too. Simply turn to the exercise section that focuses on the body part you want to reshape. Within each section you'll find a series of recommended exercises, with clear instructions on performing them correctly, as well as suggestions on exercise sequences and variations to give you the most effective muscle stimulation and thus the *fastest possible results.*

Whether you choose to work out one body part or several, it's very important you realize that this program is one of concentrated exercise. That's what it takes to get fast results. But because of the workout's concentrated nature, it's also vital you understand what you are doing and why you are doing it. *Don't just blindly jump into a routine.* First prep yourself—both mentally and physically.

36 THE MENTAL FACTOR

Your brain is one of the most powerful determinants of success in this program—probably more important even than your muscles themselves. To begin with, your brain controls your muscles—via nerve impulses sent along the neurological pathway to initiate, direct, and limit movement in a manner appropriate to the task at hand. These nerve impulses are signals telling the muscles exactly what to do, and these signals, traveling from the brain via the spinal cord, ultimately determine whether the exercise you perform is beneficial or a waste. Your brain in fact determines how strongly a muscle should contract, in what manner, and in conjunction with what other muscles. And as the muscle works, messages feed back to the brain, telling it what's happening; you feel a sensation—a "burn," a pleasing "pump" that almost verges on pain, or . . . nothing much. You also note a quickening of your breath and an acceleration of your heart rate if you sustain effort or movement over a length of time.

Everything that happens is predetermined by your brain—your mind, if you will. And that's why mental focus—concentration—is so important.

Don't waste your workouts. Think about what you are doing. Concentrate on every movement, whether you're exercising one body part or your whole body. Make that effort count! Do your exercises deliberately and purposefully, from warm-up to after-stretch.

You'll notice reminders throughout the various exercise descriptions to help you concentrate, to maintain your focus on the muscles you are working. Thinking purposefully about what you are doing will open the neurological pathways to the particular body part(s) you are perfecting. You'll find yourself automatically maintaining correct form and getting the maximum effect from each repetition.

WARMING UP

Before I explain the why of warming up, a word on what it is. I've noticed that a lot of people don't really know what it is. I must confess that, before I knew better, I used to think warming up was just a lot of unnecessary, wasted movements. Those movements didn't even "warm me up." And because I was already in pretty good shape, I thought the advice about warming up didn't apply to me . . . until I rather painfully strained the connective tissue in my shoulder joint while doing a butterfly movement (for my chest) on a machine.

That humbling experience forced me to become a beginner again while I recovered from the injury. But the rehab time turned out to be a blessing in disguise, because now I had no choice but to warm up thoroughly before *any* upper body movement. As I healed I noticed that I was able to work out more vigorously and get a much better pump in the muscle *after warming up.* (I also learned to train around my injury, applying the pain threshold principle—if it hurts, don't do it!—to my workouts.) I found myself improving, and I wasn't killing myself in the process. I learned my lesson. That was the only—and the last—injury I suffered.

A warm-up is an exercise or set of exercises that prepares your muscles for the heavy work you expect them to do later. If you simply jump into your workout routine without preparing your muscles adequately, you risk injuring yourself, even if you're in good shape.

A proper warm-up is just that—it should get your body to a point where it feels slightly warm. The warmth indicates an internal temperature increase in the muscle as a result of increased blood circulation. This prepares your body for a more vigorous exertion; it definitely helps to prevent any muscle pull or injury.

You warm up simply by moving around—vigorously. A routine series of calisthenics such as jumping jacks, running in place, jogging, or even briskly walking around will do it. Start the movement of your choice and gradually work up your speed. Continue until you feel yourself literally warming up—it can take anywhere from one to five minutes. Moving your arms vigorously in coordination with the rest of your body can cut warm-up time in half.

PRE-STRETCH

Once you feel warm, perform a pre-stretch exercise that involves the body part you are going to be exercising. This ensures proper lubrication of the joint(s) there and enables you to work the muscle through a full range of motion.

Perform the pre-stretch before your routine and, ideally, *repeat it between each set of reps.* The stretching movements send a signal to your brain that opens the neurological pathway, with the result that a greater percentage of the muscle fibers are put into play. That, of course, is what it's all about—making every rep count to its fullest and promoting flexibility at the same time.

DOING THE EXERCISES

There are anywhere from three to five exercises to perform for each body part. The number depends upon the complexity of the muscle in question. The abdominals, biceps, triceps, and calves are relatively small or simple muscle groups and need less variety for adequate stimulation, although this stimulation must still be intense to be effective. The more complex muscle groups in the chest, back, shoulders, thighs, and buttocks require more exercises; they present more of a challenge. However, if you decide to exercise complementary muscle groups, the total number of exercises required will be less than if you work the same muscles separately.

The tailor-made exercise routines given later in this chapter include isolation exercises and compound exercises, which "overlap" with respect to muscles worked.

After a light warm-up set of fifteen to twenty repetitions (these are done with less resistance than the training sets) you will do a maximum of three sets for each exercise.

And here's more good news. The weight you select for each exercise is always relative—each body part poses its own challenge and requires a different level of weight, depending on its structure and degree of development. The thigh muscles, for example, are large and can easily handle 25 pounds for a front squat, while the shoulder muscles

38

are more delicate and will find using 10- or even 5-pound dumbbells relatively difficult when doing seated side laterals. Your back will have no trouble with 40 pounds weight for the lat pull-down; your triceps will feel taxed using 5-pound dumbbells for dumbbell kickbacks.

Naturally, as your muscles grow stronger, each body part will be able to take on more resistance, but the relative differences will remain. Your thighs and back will almost always be able to handle much heavier weights than will your chest, shoulders, or triceps. Of course, the difference is individual—every woman has naturally strong and weak muscle groups.

HOW TO SELECT YOUR STARTING WEIGHTS AND NUMBER OF REPETITIONS

Here's a good rule of thumb for determining how much weight to use in any exercise: You should be able to complete a set of the particular exercise without torturing yourself *but with some difficulty.* When this is the case, your starting weight is most likely correct.

If you can complete fifteen perfect-form repetitions of any exercise without any difficulty, the weight is definitely too light. With the correct weight, you should be able to manage about ten repetitions in strict form—at least eight and not more than twelve, except when otherwise specified. (Note that the abdominals and the buttocks are in effect "special case" muscles with repetition ranges of their own—see below.)

Here's another way to determine training poundage. It's based on the maximum weight you can handle to perform an exercise in perfect form at least once. You adjust weight and number of repetitions as a percentage of the maximum. For example, if you can manage three sets of four reps with 100 pounds, you should perform three sets of at least eight reps if you are using 50 pounds for the same exercise. Some experts measure exercise intensity based on the interchangeable variables of weight and number of reps or sets—with the maximum weight that can be handled serving as the base reference point. Whether this is a good measure is still hotly debated.

Don't get obsessive about how much weight you are lifting. Your progress or potential do not primarily depend on gross weight lifted. I'm always amused to have someone ask me, "How much do you lift?" Anyone who asks that question is clearly unaware of what bodybuilding is all about.

"How much do I lift?" I ask in turn. "For which body part?"

They probably mean what maximum can I bench press or handle on a squat. But all that's beside the point. That figure only incidentally relates to how effective my exercise routine is.

Sometimes I let myself have a little fun with the question, just to see the astounded look on someone's face when I tell them, "Way over eight hundred pounds, depending on my mood." My legs are my strongest body part, especially my calves, and I can manage 800 pounds on the standing calf machine. (If it weren't that the pressure of the machine hurts the skin on my shoulders, where the resistance is applied, I could probably manage as much as 1000 pounds as a maximum repetition weight.)

People have a tendency to confuse bodybuilding with power lifting. The objectives are totally different. Power lifting has nothing to do with body esthetics. The objective is simply to lift as much poundage as possible for one "maxed-out" repetition. The objective in bodybuilding is to shape your body effectively with several sets of repetitions; the weight is a means, not an objective.

Who cares how much you can lift or how much resistance you can handle with any body part? The issue is whether you are effectively challenging your muscles to the maximum of *your* ability. If you find it a challenge to manage seven to eleven reps on your front squats with a 25-pound barbell, you'll make just as much progress as someone who finds it takes a 45-pound barbell to get that same degree of challenge. Your progress doesn't depend on the amount of weight you use, it depends on the extent to which you challenge *your* particular body part.

Even if you have a body part that's stronger than average—like me, with my calves—it isn't necessary, maybe not even desirable, to train that part heavily. Remember, you want to create a balanced effect, with body parts in perfect proportion.

INCREASING THE WEIGHT

The proper starting weight, as we've observed, is one that poses difficulty over the range of repetitions recommended for that exercise. The whole idea is giving yourself something to work *up* to. You should start with a weight that is too heavy to get twelve reps but manageable for at least eight. After anywhere from a few days to a month, you will find yourself able to manage eleven reps of the exercise with the starting weight. It's time to increase the weight, to apply the principle of "weight progression" so that you can continue your progress.

THE REP RANGE FOR ABDOMINALS

The abdominals are comparatively small muscles; they are usually underdeveloped on women and often covered with fat. As with any muscle group, in order to develop your abdominals, you have to perform appropriate exercises for a minimum number of repetitions and, if not initially, you will eventually have to use weights for added effectiveness. The rep range, however, is different from that for most other muscle groups.

You will be doing from three to five exercises for your abdominal area. As always, you will be doing three sets of repetitions for each exercise. But here's the difference: *Set a goal of twenty-five repetitions for each of the three sets of all the abdominal exercises.* Of course, you won't be able to manage that right away. Just do as many as you can and add a rep or two each week until you are up to twenty-five repetitions of each set. Then you can add light ankle weights or dumbbells to your exercises—start with 1 pound and work up to 5, or maybe even 10.

Once you are doing twenty-five reps of all the exercises for a full three sets, you can let yourself "go crazy" every once in a while: On the last set of an exercise do as many

TRY THESE ABDOMINAL COMBINATIONS

COMBINATION 1

1. **Twisting**—two minutes
2. **Crunch; oblique crunch, right side; oblique crunch, left side**—try for fifteen reps of each in sequence, then repeat the sequence a second time for two complete sets. It's better here to perform fifteen repetitions in strict form than to push for twenty-five any way you can manage them.
3. **Knee-ups**—work up to twenty-five repetitions.
4. **Leg-ups**—work up to twenty-five repetitions.
5. **Twisting**—two minutes

COMBINATION 2

1. **Twisting**—two minutes
2. **Crunch; oblique crunch, right; oblique crunch, left**—three cycles, with fifteen reps each set
3. **Knee-ups/leg-ups**—fifteen knee-ups followed by ten leg-ups for two cycles
4. **Twisting**—two minutes

COMBINATION 3

1. **Twisting**—two minutes
2. **Bent-knee leg lifts**—three sets of twenty-five reps
3. **Sit-ups**—three sets of twenty-five reps
4. **Knee-ups**—three sets of twenty-five reps
5. **Twisting**—two minutes

NOTE: The order of exercises in combinations 1 and 2 promote control, flexibility, and a full range of motion. The crunching sequence provides a very intense muscle stimulus, complemented perfectly by the knee-ups and leg-ups, which are natural stretching movements.

Be sure to include bent-knee leg lifts and sit-ups anytime you omit the crunch sequence—as here in Combination 3. Continue with knee-ups and/or leg-ups, and always finish the way you start—*twisting*.

Increase the pace of every workout. Don't hurry yourself through the exercises, however; just take less and less rest time between exercise sets.

reps as you can, just to test yourself. Who knows? You may surprise yourself by doing 200 sit-ups! Mind you, by itself this won't rid you of any fat in the stomach area, but your muscle tone and muscular endurance will be considerably improved, and you will be burning off at least some calories. And you will certainly improve your anaerobic conditioning.

REP RANGE FOR BUTTOCKS AND HIPS

Each buttock is comprised primarily of one large muscle, the gluteus maximus. The goal is to tighten and compress that muscle—to strengthen and shape it.

We do not use much in the way of weight when working the buttocks, as the primary objective is to shape and lift it rather than build mass. However, to accomplish that we do have to keep the number of reps high and work the muscle intensely.

There are four different exercises for the buttocks. *Aim for twenty-five repetitions for all three sets of each exercise.* Of course, you probably won't be able to get twenty-five reps for each set at the beginning. Just do as many as you can, and add two reps each week until you have worked up to three sets of twenty-five reps for each exercise.

Once you manage the full twenty-five reps for all sets, add 1-pound ankle weights on each leg. When you can again do twenty-five reps on all three sets, add another pound on each ankle, and continue this weight progression until you are using 5 pounds on each ankle.

HOW OFTEN SHOULD YOU WORK OUT?

If you are working anywhere from one to four body parts, the best schedule generally is to work out three days a week, alternating workout days with rest days. How you schedule your three workout days depends on your situation. You may choose to work out Monday, Wednesday, and Friday or Tuesday, Thursday, and Saturday.

When working out a single body part, just follow the suggested order of exercises given for that part. The exercises indicated include both "compound movements" and "isolation movements," which in combination assure you balanced development of the particular body part. Compound movements are those that not only exercise the major muscle(s) you are focusing on but also smaller muscles that work in a complementary manner to accomplish those movements. Isolation movements primarily work the major muscle(s) you are concerned with. In some cases, particularly when working the calves, you depend on a mixture of isolation exercises, since it's not as easy to work the muscles that comprise that body part equally all at one time.

The table here provides a summary of compound and isolation exercises for different body parts:

42

COMPOUND AND ISOLATION EXERCISES

Body Part	Secondary Muscle(s)	Compound Exercise	Isolation Exercise
Chest	Triceps	Dumbbell presses	Hand-on-knee isometric concentrations
	Lats	Cross bench pull-overs	Isometric contractions Flyes Cable crossovers Pec deck
Triceps	(You will be using your forearms to some degree, but the exercises here will not actually work the muscles there to the extent of serving as compound exercises.)		Cross-face triceps extensions Dumbbell kickbacks Pulley push-downs Two-arm dumbbell extensions
Shoulders	Triceps	Alternating dumbbell presses	Pee Wee laterals Side laterals Bent-over laterals
	Trapezius, biceps	Upright rows	
Abdomen	Lower back, thighs	Standard sit-ups	Crunches
	Hip flexors	Knee-ups on bench	
	Thighs	Straight leg lifts on bench	
	Hip flexors, thighs	Bent-knee leg lifts Knee-tuck leg raiser combination	
Hips/buttocks	Hamstrings, lower back	Standing hip hyperextensions	Pelvic lifts Single/double-leg buttocks tighteners

Spot training is a great concept, but fortunately God created a wonderful piece of machinery comprised of elements that work together in harmony. So even though you may concentrate your energies on developing specific body parts in isolation, you'll experience a wider benefit. You'll be toning the complementary muscles at the same time.

Combining compound and isolation movements in the sequences presented here will automatically bring into play an intensification technique that leads to balanced muscle development. You'll find isolation movements will *pre-exhaust* the target muscle(s); then the combination movements will push them to the point of failure while

COMPOUND AND ISOLATION EXERCISES

Body Part	Secondary Muscle(s)	Compound Exercise	Isolation Exercise
	Medial glutes, thighs, lower back, hips	Lunges	
Thighs	Medial glutes, inner thigh, outer buttock	Bugs Bunny lunges	Leg curls Leg extensions Sissy squats
	Buttocks, lower back	Front squats Leg presses Lunges	
Back	Thighs, forearms	Dead lifts	Straight-arm body pulls
	Biceps, forearms	Lat pull-downs to the rear/front	
	Biceps, rear delts	Pulley rows Barbell bent rows	
	Biceps, rear delts, trapezius	One-/two-arm dumbbell rows	
Biceps	(Anytime you grip, you automatically bring the forearms into play to some degree, but not to the extent that the exercises serve a combination purpose.)		Standing alternate dumbbell curls Angled dumbbell curls Standing barbell curls
Calves	(There are no combination exercises here, and some of the isolation movements actually work only a section of calf muscle, e.g., the soleus or gastrocnemius.)		Seated calf raises Standing calf machine presses Seated dumbbell calf raises Single-leg calf raises Rotational calf raises

bringing complementary muscles into play at the same time. (Stimulating muscles to further development requires working them to the limits of their capabilities—your muscles won't feel a need to develop further if the demands you make of them are easily within their current capabilities.)

If you are working two body parts that complement each other naturally, you can in fact take advantage of their complementary nature and plan a *combination routine.* That is because you will already be bringing the second group of muscles into play while working the first group, and you'll continue working the first group as you move onto exercises that primarily target the second group. In other instances you can work two body parts effectively in combination by *supersetting*, performing a set for one part and immediately following with a set for the other part, in effect combining the two sets into a continuous super set that exercises both body parts. The total number of sets you perform will still be the same, but where previously you might have performed three sets of exercises for one body part and then followed with three sets of exercises for the next body part, now you do three combination super sets. (You can also superset two exercises for the same body part.)

When working out more than one body part, the order of your exercises can make a difference. In particular, you should *never* train your chest, back, or shoulders *after* training your arms. Your arms come into play in all the exercises for the chest, back, and shoulders, and if you first work your arms separately to the point of exhaustion, then when it comes to working out the larger muscle groups, your arms will simply give out before you can stimulate the other muscles sufficiently to affect development.

Your calves can be trained with just about any other body part, since they are exercised in relative isolation. They are stimulated to a fair extent when you perform a leg workout, particularly when doing leg curls, so it makes sense to train them *after* a general leg workout.

SUGGESTED COMBINATION ROUTINES

Back and biceps. Do the full back routine as given, then finish off your biceps with two exercises of your choice. The standing alternate dumbbell curl supersetted with the angled dumbbell curl would be a good choice.

Chest and triceps. Complete the chest routine as given, then finish with just the first two triceps exercises. Your triceps will have been sufficiently stimulated in doing the chest movements to make the balance of the triceps exercises unnecessary.

Triceps and biceps. Include all the movements given in the routines for these muscles, but combine them in super sets. Try these sequences:

- **In the gym:** pulley push-downs supersetted with either barbell curls or angled dumbbell curls, then seated two-arm dumbbell extensions supersetted with alternate dumbbell curls, and finish with cross-face dumbbell extensions.
- **At home:** seated two-arm dumbbell extensions supersetted with barbell curls, kickbacks supersetted with alternate dumbbell curls or angled dumbbell curls, finishing off with cross-face triceps extensions.

Chest and shoulders. Do the complete chest routine. After a warm-up set for the shoulders, continue with three sets of side laterals, Pee Wee laterals, *or* bent-over laterals. The chest workout will have stimulated the frontal deltoids sufficiently so that all you need to do for a complete shoulder routine is stimulate the medial and rear heads of the deltoids with one or other of the lateral exercises.

Chest, shoulders, and triceps. Follow the same routine as for the chest and shoulders combination and add the same two triceps movements indicated for the chest and triceps combination (cross-face triceps extensions and two-arm dumbbell extensions).

Abdominals, back, shoulders, and chest. The muscles that flex the torso work in conjunction with those that produce spinal movement. They operate in pairs—a pair running on either side of the spinal column in the back and paired muscles in the abdomen. When you exercise your abdominals, you necessarily also work the muscles of your lower back. This makes an abdominal workout the perfect way to warm up the lower back area (although you will still need to do a warm-up set for the upper back if you decide on this combination).

Complete the routine for your abdominals as given, continue with the exercises for your back. Then reverse the order of exercises recommended for the chest and shoulder combination—do the laterals, then finish with the chest routine.

Chest and back. This is a popular combination, but you will still have to perform all the exercises given. The difference is that you can either perform the routines as suggested or superset the chest exercises with the back exercises.

Chest, shoulders, and back. Follow the directions for the chest and shoulders combination, then finish with only three additional movements for the back in the gym: lat pull-downs, pulley rows, and one-arm dumbbell rows. At home finish with one-arm bent rows, seated dumbbell back laterals, straight-arm body pulls, and *one set* of deadlifts. The shoulder muscles flow into the back muscles, so this progression of exercises is a natural combination.

Full upper body workout. To the above combination, add the first two triceps exercises and two biceps movements. (The biceps will already have been stimulated in doing the back exercises.) Try alternating a triceps movement with a biceps movement when finishing up your arms. The combination routine for the entire upper body should take *less* than an hour! Go ahead and finish off your workout with a few abdominal exercises just for the fun of it!

Thighs and buttocks. Do just the first three exercises in the routines given for these two body parts, buttocks first. You can omit the rest!

SAMPLE COMBINATION ROUTINES

AT HOME	IN THE GYM

Thighs and buttocks

AT HOME	IN THE GYM
Leg curls	Leg curls
Front squats	Front squats
Lunges	Lunges
Standing hip hyperextensions	
Pelvic lifts	
Buttocks tightener	

Chest and triceps

AT HOME	IN THE GYM
Incline flyes	Incline flyes
Dumbbell presses	Pec deck
Isometric contractions	Cable crossovers
Cross-bench pullovers	Pullovers
Cross-face triceps extensions	Cross-face triceps extensions
Two-arm dumbbell extensions	Press-downs or two-arm dumbbell extensions

Chest and shoulders

AT HOME	IN THE GYM
Incline flyes	Incline flyes
Dumbbell presses	Pec deck
Isometric contractions	Cable crossovers
Cross-bench pullovers	Pullovers
Side laterals	Side laterals
Bent-over or Pee Wee laterals	Bent-over or Pee Wee laterals

Chest, shoulders, triceps

AT HOME	IN THE GYM
Incline flyes	Incline flyes
Dumbbell presses	Pec deck
Isometric contractions	Cable crossovers
Cross-bench pullovers	Pullovers
Side laterals	Side laterals
Bent-over or Pee Wee laterals	Bent-over or Pee Wee laterals
Cross-face triceps extensions	Cross-face triceps extensions
Two-arm triceps extensions	Push-downs or two-arm triceps extensions

Chest, shoulders, back

Incline flyes	Incline flyes
Dumbbell presses	Pec deck
Isometric contractions	Cable crossovers
Cross-bench pullovers	Pullovers
Side laterals	Side laterals
Pee Wee laterals	Pee Wee laterals
One-arm bent rows	Lat pull-downs
Seated dumbbell back laterals	Pulley rows
Straight-arm body pulls	One-arm dumbbell rows

Entire upper body (chest, shoulders, back, arms)

To the exercises for the chest, shoulders, and back add:

Cross-face dumbbell extensions, supersetted with two-arm triceps extensions	Push-downs, supersetted with standing barbell curls
Standing barbell curls, supersetted with alternate dumbbell curls	Cross-face triceps extensions, supersetted with alternate dumbbell curls

SPLIT ROUTINES

If you decide to work on more than four body parts, your best option is probably to go onto a schedule of split routines, which leads to remarkable results.

On the split routine, you will work out four days a week, exercising half your body on workout days one and three, the other half on workout days two and four. Split routines allow for a flexible approach to body shaping. You can change routines from week to week according to your sense of what combination of exercises works best for you. You might choose to split your routines in the following manner:

- **Workout days one and three**—chest, shoulders, triceps, and abdominals
- **Workout days two and four**—buttocks, thighs, back, biceps, calves

If you feel your buttocks and abdominals need extra attention, then separately work them on a fifth day, as they require more stimulation to develop optimally. Performing the exercises for those two body parts alone should take you about twenty-five minutes.

When on a split routine, you can still eliminate overlapping exercises by following the combination routines indicated above. Once you've mastered the exercises, it should take you no more than an hour to do a complete workout (but you should never race the clock when performing your exercises).

48

CIRCUIT WEIGHT TRAINING

One of the complaints about weight training is that it is not *aerobic* and so does not benefit the cardiovascular system the way that exercises like running, sustained calisthenics, or swimming laps do. As we've already observed, to burn fat off most efficiently also takes getting into an aerobic mode.

The fact is that weight training can provide aerobic benefits as well as strength and muscle development, but this means adapting your routine so that you perform your exercises with a minimum of rest in between. The best way to manage this is through circuit training—doing sets of exercises in rapid succession through the whole circuit of your routine. Do twelve to fifteen reps of each exercise, then move on to the next exercise immediately, without taking time to rest. I recommend this kind of workout occasionally—whenever you really want to energize yourself for a real charge or when you just can't fit aerobic exercises into your schedule but still want a concentrated workout.

A QUICK FULL-BODY WORKOUT CIRCUIT

For a simple circuit routine, perform just the exercises indicated in the column to the left. For super circuit weight training, superset the indicated exercise on the left with the exercise on the corresponding line in the column on the right.

Crunches	_____
Twisting	_____
Bent-over rows	Two-arm dumbbell rows
Deadlifts	Stiff-legged deadlifts
Alternate dumbbell curls	Angled dumbbell curls
Incline/decline chest flyes	Presses
Side laterals	Alternate dumbbell presses
Two-arm dumbbell extensions	Dumbbell kickbacks
Pelvic lifts with weight on hip	_____
Lunges	Squats

BREAKING IN SLOWLY

49

If you've never exercised before, all this may sound too complex and strenuous to undertake, however much you'd like to see the promised results. Well, you don't have to start with everything at once. Focus on one to three body parts, and break in slowly. Follow the appropriate diet given in chapter 16 at the same time, particularly if you are overweight.

Here's a four-week break-in plan:

- **Week one:** Do only the warm-up/pre-stretch and a warm-up set of fifteen to twenty reps for each exercise.
- **Week two:** Do the warm-up/pre-stretch, a warm-up set of fifteen to twenty reps, and one regular set of seven to eleven reps for each exercise.
- **Week three:** Do the warm-up/pre-stretch, a warm-up set of fifteen to twenty repetitions, and two regular sets of from seven to eleven reps for each exercise.
- **Week four:** Do the warm-up/pre-stretch, the warm-up set of fifteen to twenty reps, and all three sets of seven to eleven reps for each exercise.

This is a good break-in system, whether you are working just one body part or your whole body.

Give yourself time to get used to working out. At first it may seem there's a lot to learn, that there's a big adjustment to make. The important thing is not to give up. Breaking in slowly allows you time to learn the movements and time to make the necessary adjustment to a regular exercise routine.

You will see results. I guarantee it. Even if you start with just one body part, you'll be delighted with the changes the mirror reflects back to you in as little as three months time. You may suddenly find that you have the time to fit a whole body workout into your very busy schedule once you realize the power you have to reshape and revitalize yourself.

Go for it!

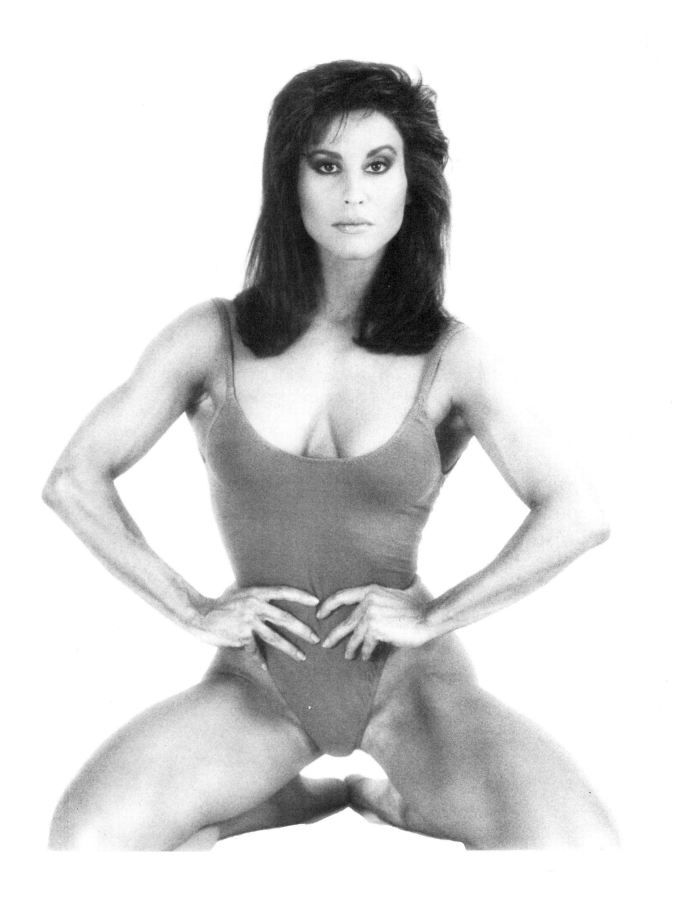

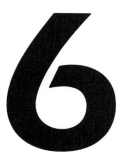

6

Body Perfection Techniques

When shaping your body, the same principle applies as in any other area of personal endeavor: To get what you want, you have to go about it the right way. And you start by making up your mind that you *are* going to get what you want.

In this chapter you'll learn the different perfection techniques that put having that perfect body you want within closer reach. In all of them the focus is on effectively maximizing *intensity of contraction*, because that's at the heart of stimulating muscle development. It boils down to a matter of physical excellence.

EXERCISE FORM

Some of the techniques that follow are options, but there's no option on exercise form if you want your workouts to count. Correct form can mean the difference between a beneficial workout and a wasted one. Sloppy form doesn't do your muscles a bit of good. It wastes your time and invites injury.

So what is good exercise form?

Well, first let me tell you what it isn't. It isn't throwing, swinging, or jerking movements. These should be avoided at all costs, or they'll cost you—and maybe plenty!

Good form requires that the entire exercise movement for every repetition be performed in a smooth, deliberate style. And pay special attention to the lowering or second half of the movement.

Don't let any other part of your body help in a movement designed for a specific muscle or muscle group. That's called "cheating." Move the target muscle(s) through the full range of motion in each exercise—to the full degree of extension, to the full degree of contraction, and then back again. This full range of motion in combination with the proper stance or body position for the exercise is what correct form is all about.

CONTINUOUS TENSION

Maintaining continuous tension throughout an exercise is not really a special technique. For the most part, this is just an elaboration on correct exercise form. Ideally, you should maintain continuous tension through each rep of each set of every exercise.

The reminder to maintain continuous tension is given here simply because it's so tempting and easy to forget to do that. It's an unfortunate human trait to try to short-cut any effort that entails some degree of difficulty. If you do that with body shaping exercises, you won't get the body shaping effect they are designed to provide.

Continuous tension means just that. You keep tension on the working muscle(s) at all times. You do not let momentum rob you of even a split second of contraction intensity, because that precious sustained contraction is what gives you results—with each rep. There are special intensification techniques you can choose as options, but there's no option here if you want your workouts to count.

PEAK CONTRACTION

You receive the greatest benefit from an exercise repetition when the maximum number of muscle cells are contracted to their maximum load capability—that is, worked against the greatest resistance they can handle. With peak contraction, the muscle is exerted to its fullest extent in a completely contracted (flexed) position.

If you're familiar with weight training, you'll realize almost immediately that you don't get a peak contraction with some bodybuilding exercises—there's little or virtually no stress on the muscle when it's in a fully contracted position. A good example is the standing barbell curl. When you've curled the barbell up to the point where your biceps are fully contracted, there's relatively little resistance directly on the muscle.

Here's where Nautilus machines provide an advantage—you always get maximum resistance on a contracted muscle. But there are many exercises using free weights that also give you a peak contraction effect—all calf exercises, leg extensions, most leg curls, all pulley push- or pull-downs, side laterals, front laterals, bent-over laterals, dumbbell kickbacks, and rowing movements, among others.

I've also noticed that while some machines help you achieve a peak contraction in the fully flexed position, they are too easy at the beginning of a movement. What you gain at one point you lose at another. Peak contraction isn't the only determining factor in muscle development. And peak contraction won't make a difference if it isn't preceded—and followed—by continuous tension while maintaining perfect form.

MUSCLE CONTRACTION SPECIFICITY

Okay. Say you're doing your set. You've got perfect exercise form, you're feeling continuous tension throughout each movement, and you can even feel the achievement of a peak contraction. What next?

What I do is go beyond perfection at this point. (I can hear you telling yourself, "She must be nuts!") I apply what I call the principle of muscle contraction specificity.

In shaping muscle, you can do more than simply stimulate its overall development. You can actually predetermine how its shape develops. You do so by adjusting the exercise movement to shift the point of maximum stress to where you want to see the most development. A slight shift in your body position or a slight twist of angle will make all the difference between a regular peak contraction and a peak contraction with purpose.

I can't give you a scientific explanation here; I have no outside authorities to cite in support of this special developmental technique. I can only tell you I have found that it works for me and has worked for others I've shared it with. Again, the important thing is to maintain good form and continuous tension. The change in form is calculated; don't try kidding yourself that careless or sloppy form—poor stance and bad angles—will get you the same results.

I've found that buttocks lifting exercises (for example, pelvic lifts done either the regular way or with one leg up, buttocks tighteners, and lunges with a buttocks squeeze) lend themselves to the slight modification that gives muscle contraction specificity. I'm convinced that slightly shifting body position in these exercises affects the shape of the lift you are working for. The whole philosophy behind *Perfect Parts* is that you can achieve the shape that's right for you. The point isn't just to build muscles for the sake of having muscles.

BURNS

After a few months of consistent training, many people turn to specialized techniques to intensify their workouts and consequently get quicker, better results. Doing "burns" is one of the more popular of those techniques. But read through the following description carefully before deciding on this technique for yourself, and use your best judgment with regard to your readiness to try burns.

Burns are quick, partial reps done at the end of the last repetition of your normal set. These quick, partial reps force your muscle(s) to keep working past the point at which you would normally experience failure using correct form. (Failure simply refers to a muscle's inability to perform a next rep after reaching the point of exhaustion.)

The reason these partial reps are called burns is because they burn! The sensation is caused by an abnormally high buildup of lactic acid in the working muscle tissue, which the blood cannot carry away fast enough.

But consider this: If the blood cannot carry away this waste product, it probably cannot bring in sufficient fresh oxygen to replenish the muscle promptly either. I don't know about you, but I do not particularly like the idea that I may be suffocating my muscles. And I am not altogether convinced that my muscles would appreciate my forcing them in this way, especially when they've already been trained to failure while maintaining strict exercise form with continuous tension. Then too, these are just partial reps, which means I would *not* be maintaining correct form through a full range of motion, and that's something I'm not eager to endorse.

Here's my point: Be wary of anyone telling you to adopt a special technique that entails dropping correct form and compounds muscle failure with some kind of pain. First of all, it isn't necessary. The "burn" is no indication that your muscles are being stimulated in a manner that leads to more rapid development. If burn was such a magic factor, then every woman who has ever followed those exercise video tapes (you know which ones I'm talking about) would be a shining example of tight, shapely femininity. I know lots of women who "burned" their way through video exercise routines and never saw much in the way of improvement in their shape.

To my mind, burns are excessive. To quote Arthur Jones, designer of the Nautilus exercise machines, "It takes only one properly placed, or 'correct' shot to kill a rabbit or an elephant. Additional shots will serve no purpose except unnecessary destruction of flesh."

Think about it! No amount of improper stimulation will ever give you worthwhile results. Besides, you don't need to torture your muscles to get noticeable results. Exercise can and should be a gratifying experience, accomplished with a sense of respect for your body.

TRAINING PAST FAILURE

A basic principle in weight (resistance) training is working the target muscle(s) through a full range of movement until you can't complete another full repetition under your own power. All the exercise routines given here are designed to bring you to that point of "failure." It sounds awful, but don't let the term scare you off. It's nothing more than bodybuilding lingo used to identify a certain aspect of exercise activity. Basically, the principle is simply to challenge muscle to the limits of its capabilities, because that's what it takes to move beyond those limits.

But if training to failure means pushing yourself to the limit of your capabilities, then how can you talk of training past failure?

It's really quite simple. You do one of two things. Either you no longer rely entirely on your own muscle power to complete additional reps once you've reached your point of failure, or you force out a few additional reps without maintaining strict form once you've reached your point of failure while adhering to strict form. Doing burns is in fact one way of training past failure, but not a technique I recommend. Two techniques that I have found to be effective when done properly are "cheating" and "forced reps."

Cheating. When we talk about cheating in bodybuilding, we mean performing an exercise with less than perfect form. As an effective technique, however, that's limited to a very specific set of circumstances.

Cheating throughout an exercise set means you are reducing stress on a muscle or muscle group that you must stress to the maximum in order to prompt development. Cheating as a technique for training past failure means something else altogether—it means maintaining maximum sustainable stress on a muscle that first has been trained to failure while adhering to perfect form. You're actually continuing the exercise past the point where you'd otherwise stop—you're adding stress, not removing it. You are, however, sacrificing form at that point.

Say you've taken a set of alternating dumbbell curls to failure with 15 pounds. That means you can't do another rep in perfect form with those 15 pounds. It doesn't mean you can't manage, say, 10 pounds. The objective of cheating is to introduce *just enough* extraneous body movement to allow the weight resistance to continue stimulating the muscle beyond the point where it would normally fail.

Proper cheating (yes, it does sound a little funny) entails exerting just enough pressure with other muscles or through body movement to get the weight up past your sticking point and then lowering it *slowly.* (It's important to resist the downward motion, not to just let the weight drop of its own accord.)

More than two or three cheats will be futile. Also, I recommend that you not use this technique until you have mastered training to failure in perfect style for at least six months.

Forced reps. Here, too, we're talking about one to three extra reps once you've worked the target muscle(s) to failure. But in this case you rely on an outside source of assistance—a regular training partner preferably—rather than cheat on form of movement.

This is a more precise technique for lessening weight resistance once you've hit your sticking point. Your training partner *spots* you, standing close by—right over you in some cases—to pull up on or otherwise slightly lessen the weight resistance once you reach failure. Naturally, you want a training partner who can read exactly when and how much to assist you on a forced rep. That's why a regular training partner who knows you and is familiar with your routine works best.

Here again, more than two or three reps will be unproductive. Unlike cheating, however, you should always maintain proper form. A good training partner, in fact, will act not only as a spotter but remind you to adhere to proper form anytime you show a tendency to cheat.

56 SUPER SETS AND GIANT SETS

At the heart of the exercise program here are repetitions of movements done in sets. As we've noted, a repetition is simply a single complete exercise movement. A set is a number of repetitions of the same movement performed without a rest break. Most standard sets include from eight to twelve reps, although abdominal and buttocks exercise sets may include as many as twenty-five reps.

When we speak of straight sets, we mean nothing more than two to three sets of the same movement, one after the other, usually with a brief rest interval between each set. (The rest interval allows the target muscle or muscle group to recuperate just enough to complete the following set adequately.) If you are just beginning weight training, I recommend you stick to straight sets for at least the first twelve weeks of training.

Super sets. A super set is the combination of two sets of two different exercises with a shorter than normal, if any, rest period between the two combined sets, although a normal rest interval will be needed between the super sets.

Super sets intensify your workout. You can superset exercises for different body parts—for example, a triceps movement with a biceps movement, a quadriceps movement with a hamstrings movement, or a chest movement with a back movement. Working two antagonistic muscle groups together like this is the least intense form of supersetting, but it is still effective and can save time.

A more intense form of supersetting is to combine two sets of different exercises for the same body part. For example, the *Perfect Parts* biceps routine recommends supersetting alternate dumbbell curls with angled dumbbell curls. Warm up first as suggested in the exercise description, then perform your first set of alternate dumbbell curls. After you perform the last rep in that set, go directly into a set of angled dumbbell curls. Make sure there is as little rest time as possible between the two exercise sets, and don't sacrifice correct exercise form in moving from one set to the other. After the super set, you'll need about a minute's time to allow your biceps to recover sufficiently to be able to perform a next super set. At the end of the second super set, take a minute to recover, then finish off with one or two sets of standing barbell curls. (If you've performed the super sets with correct form, it's unlikely you'll be able to manage three sets of the curls.)

Pre-exhaustion super sets. Certain exercises work a muscle in relative isolation, while other exercises work both the target muscle and others that act in a complementary fashion to make a particular movement possible. The former are termed isolation exercises, the latter compound exercises. (See the chart in chapter 5 for a listing of isolation and compound exercises for different body parts.)

With pre-exhaustion super sets, what you do is first work a target muscle to failure with an isolation exercise, then move to a compound exercise that works the muscle in conjunction with others to perform the specified movement *without intervening rest time*. Bringing the other muscles into play in the compound movement provides just enough difference so that the target muscle, "pre-exhausted" by the isolation set, can continue to perform. It's something like a set of forced reps, except that instead of a training partner assisting on the movement to keep you going, other muscles provide the assistance.

It's important that you not approach this like two separate sets, with a rest period in between. The movements should segue naturally in what amounts to one continuous series—a single super set. Once again the objective is to train past failure, which provides an extra degree of stimulus to muscle growth.

Here are some sample pre-exhaustion superset combinations. The first movement given is the isolation exercise; the second is the compound exercise.

- **For the chest:** incline flyes plus incline presses; pec deck plus pressing movements
- **For the abdominals:** crunches plus knee-ups
- **For the shoulders:** side laterals plus alternate dumbbell presses
- **For the back:** pullovers plus lat pull-downs
- **For the buttocks:** weighted pelvic lifts plus lunges with buttocks squeeze
- **For the thighs:** leg extensions plus front squats

While pre-exhaustion super sets are a very effective way of intensifying a workout of a particular body part, that does not mean you should train like this on a regular basis. Rather the purpose of these combinations is to interject intensity into your workouts periodically to keep your muscles stimulated in such a way that they continue to improve in development.

Giant sets. When you combine three or more exercises with little or no rest between movements, then you are performing a tri-set (if just three) or giant set. Giant sets are more difficult than doing regular super sets, but they are an excellent way to thoroughly train muscles that need stimulation from different angles in order to develop optimally. The deltoids are an example of such a muscle. You need to stimulate the anterior, medial, and posterior heads to get even development.

Here's what a giant set for the shoulders might look like:

1. Side laterals
2. Pee Wee laterals
3. Upright rows
4. Bent-over laterals

You perform the exercises in this sequence with little or no rest between movements. You take a rest only upon finishing the complete series, then you repeat the sequence in another continuous run-through.

PYRAMID SETS

58

Many bodybuilders adopt a pyramid system of sets to stimulate a muscle or muscle group to the maximum. What this entails is adding weight to successive sets of a movement until you reach a peak, then decreasing weights successively on the downside until you are at your starting weight.

Here's how it might work with seated alternate biceps curls:

Set 1: twelve repetitions with 5 pounds
Set 2: ten repetitions with 10 pounds
Set 3: six to eight repetitions with 15 pounds
Set 4: five to seven repetitions with 10 pounds
Set 5: four to six repetitions with 5 pounds

You don't simply lower the weights once you've reached the peak because it's a pyramid and you're supposed to. You lower them because once you've reached that peak effort you can't possibly do another set without lowering the weights—or the second set thereafter without lowering them again. Note that the number of reps decreases at each step, reflecting the growing exhaustion of the targeted muscles.

Pyramiding weights ensures maximum muscular challenge. The progressive change in intensity forces your muscle to continual adjustment and development.

You can apply the pyramid system to any set of exercises performed with weight. It can't be applied to abdominal and buttocks exercises that do not entail the use of weights.

Modified pyramid sets. In the modified pyramid system, you add weight to each set of the exercise and decrease the number of repetitions until you reach your peak. Then you stop. You do not descend with further sets of progressively decreased weight.

This method is used by most champion bodybuilders as a regular part of their routine. It eliminates training boredom and encourages you to reach for maximum intensity. Decreasing the rest time between sets further adds to the intensity.

It's a good idea to switch to the pyramid system if you find yourself getting bored with performing straight sets using the same weight. However, when you switch to a pyramid system—the modified pyramid is better as a start—be careful not to waste that first set by selecting too light a weight. Your first set should consist of twelve to fifteen repetitions using a weight that forces you to work *hard* to make the full number of reps.

Here's an example of a modified pyramid series when doing seated alternate concentration curls:

Set 1: twelve to fifteen repetitions with 10 pounds
Set 2: eight to ten repetitions with 15 pounds
Set 3: six to eight repetitions with 20 pounds

Remember to raise your weights progressively once completing the pyramid becomes too easy. When you first do so, you will probably find that you can't manage quite as many reps at each step. However, in a month or so you are likely to find these increased weights too easy as well. That means it's time to raise the weights again.

CHOOSING A SPECIAL PERFECTION TECHNIQUE

After you've established a regular exercise routine over a period of several months, it's a good idea to incorporate one or two of the special perfection techniques into your training for a month or two. Then eliminate those and try another one or two, and so on until you have experimented with all of them. You may find you decide to incorporate a particular technique—maybe two of them—into your regular training routine.

But keep this in account, too. The human body adapts remarkably well to any routine, including a routine of stress—in this case, purposeful physical stress. Your muscles can get used to the same routine repeated over and over. After a while they don't respond to that too familiar stimulus with further development. That's why it's important to introduce variations in your routine periodically—to keep your muscles "off balance," to force them to make unexpected adjustments and thus keep improving.

As you become more and more aware of your body's response to the stimulus of exercise, you'll find yourself taking advantage of different techniques at different times. Just don't forget that the purpose of changes in your routine is to increase the intensity—*the quality of effort* directed toward making your workout work for you.

Let your body guide you. Learn to tune into your particular needs. No two bodies are alike; what works best for me or another woman won't necessarily work best for you. Give yourself time to make adjustments. Soon these things will become natural to you. By the time you've been training a year you'll feel like an expert.

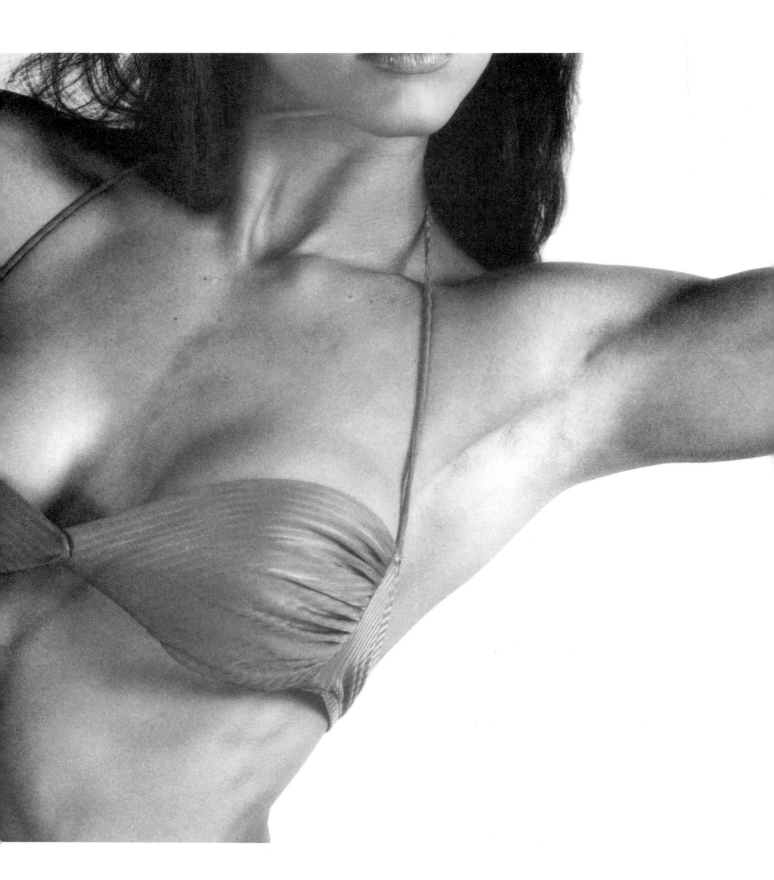

7

The *Perfect Parts* Chest Routine

A woman's chest has always been the focus of attention. Your chest muscles, which give lift and add shape to your breasts, are properly called "pectoral muscles." Well-developed pectoral muscles contribute to a perfectly balanced body.

Many women express fear of working out their chest muscles. "Will I lose my breasts?" or "Won't I get too big if I work my chest with weights?" are typical questions I hear from worried women. Stop worrying! If you work out with weights, you will *not* lose your breasts. You will instead form an attractive line of cleavage, which is one of the most appealing forms of definition found on the feminine physique. You will *not* get "too big." Rather you will develop firm, uplifted breasts, which would otherwise begin to sag with time as the force of gravity takes its toll. Firm muscles formed under your breasts counteract the downward pull of time.

Every woman should work her chest, whether she is large-breasted or small-breasted. A small-breasted woman will develop cleavage, and that definition will cause her breasts to appear larger and more shapely. A large-breasted woman will develop firm muscles under her breasts, resulting in a firm, uplifted look. In either case, the overall effect is one of perfection.

The pectoral muscles are located just under your breasts. They are not there just for esthetic reasons. They function to help you move your arms. The muscles are shaped like fans and spread from your collarbone to your breastbone. The pectorals are actually divided into two areas, upper (clavicular) and medial (sternal). Your upper

61

62

pectoral muscles are smaller than your medial pectoral muscles, but they require exercise, too, in order to create a perfectly balanced pectoral or breast area. I have included specific exercises for the entire area of your pectoral muscles.

DEVELOPMENT

In terms of speed of development, the pectoral muscles are usually somewhere in the middle. They neither jump into shape nor do they lag behind. However, your particular pectoral development will depend upon your genetic makeup. You may develop more quickly or a little bit more slowly than others. Expect to feel an uplifting tightness after a few workouts and to see some visible results between three weeks and two months.

If you are extremely overweight, chances are your breasts are holding some of your excess fat. As you begin working out and dieting, your breasts will begin both to lose excess fat and to develop firm muscle. Don't panic if at first they seem to be getting smaller. In the long run they will look firmer, tighter, and more perfectly formed. They will not appear significantly smaller, unless, of course, you were extremely overweight, and then the amount of size you lost will be made up for in the quality of your new breasts.

EXERCISES

There are five exercises for your chest workout. Here is the list. If you are working at home, follow the home list. If you are working in the gym, follow the gym list.

HOME CHEST ROUTINE

1. Incline dumbbell flye
2. Flat dumbbell press
3. Cross-bench pullover
4. Hand-on-knee isometric contractions *plus* variation
5. Flat dumbbell flye

GYM CHEST ROUTINE

1. Incline dumbbell flye
2. Pec deck flye
3. Cable crossover
4. Cross-bench pullover
5. Flat dumbbell flye

The home chest routine is presented first. The gym workout follows that. But before you begin, read the instructions regarding warm-ups and repetitions and weights.

After completing your warm-up do seven to eleven repetitions for each of your three sets. If you find that you cannot get at least seven repetitions for your set, you have selected too heavy a weight. If you find that you're getting eleven repetitions too easily, you have selected too light a weight. And don't forget to raise your weight once it gets too easy (after about a month, we'd estimate—everyone is different).

HOW OFTEN TO WORK OUT

63

See chapter 5 for details. If you are working only your chest or your chest and another body part or two, you should work *every other day* or *three times a week*. If you have chosen to do your entire body, follow the four-day split routine described in chapter 5, which would work your chest twice a week.

WARM-UP/PRE-STRETCH

Clasp your hands behind your lower back and slowly straighten your arms (your hands will be away from your body). This will stretch your chest muscles. Hold the stretch for a slow count to five, then repeat.

Next stand in the middle of a doorway or next to a sturdy upright pole or pillar. Take a giant step forward. While looking straight ahead, reach back with your right arm, turning the palm of your hand away from your body. Bracing yourself against the doorway or pole with your outstretched hand, twist your body slightly to the left. Feel the stretch in the right side of your chest and hold for a few seconds. Repeat the movement, and then stretch the opposite side in the same way.

As well as using this as a warm-up, repeat the movement at the end of your chest workout. Remember to perform fifteen reps as a preliminary warm-up set.

64 HOME CHEST ROUTINE

Incline Dumbbell Flye

This is my favorite chest exercise. It perfects the upper pectoral (breast) muscles. It helps to develop a full, high cleavage and to give the breasts a firmer, higher look. It also provides indirect stimulation to the frontal deltoids and triceps.

POSITIONING

- Hold a dumbbell in each hand and lie with your back flat against the incline exercise bench.
- With your palms facing each other, extend your arms straight up so that the dumbbells are directly above your shoulder joints at full arm's length.
- Hold the dumbbells in alignment with each other, so that the outer part of your wrists face each other. This gives you a much better contraction.

THE MOVEMENT

- Slightly bend your arms and extend them downward in a semicircular movement until you feel a complete stretch in your upper pectoral (chest) area. Keeping your upper back flat against the bench, take a deep breath and push your chest slightly outward to get the full stretch.

- Exhale forcefully as you bring the dumbbells back to start position and flex (squeeze together) your pectoral muscles.

- Repeat the movement until you have completed your set.

REMEMBER

- Stretch on every down movement and flex on every up movement.
- Don't hold your breath.
- Keep your mind focused on your chest muscles and really push your chest into this movement. Your chest is supposed to be doing the work. Think of your arms as mere "handles" or levers to hold the weights.
- Beware of the temptation to let your back rise too much from the back of the bench. This happens if the weight is too heavy. If you cannot keep your back nearly flat on the bench and perform the movement correctly, lower your weights. In time you will be strong enough to increase your weights. Performing the exercise incorrectly will only result in haphazard and miniscule development.
- Picture your breasts being shaped and uplifted as you perform the exercise.

Start

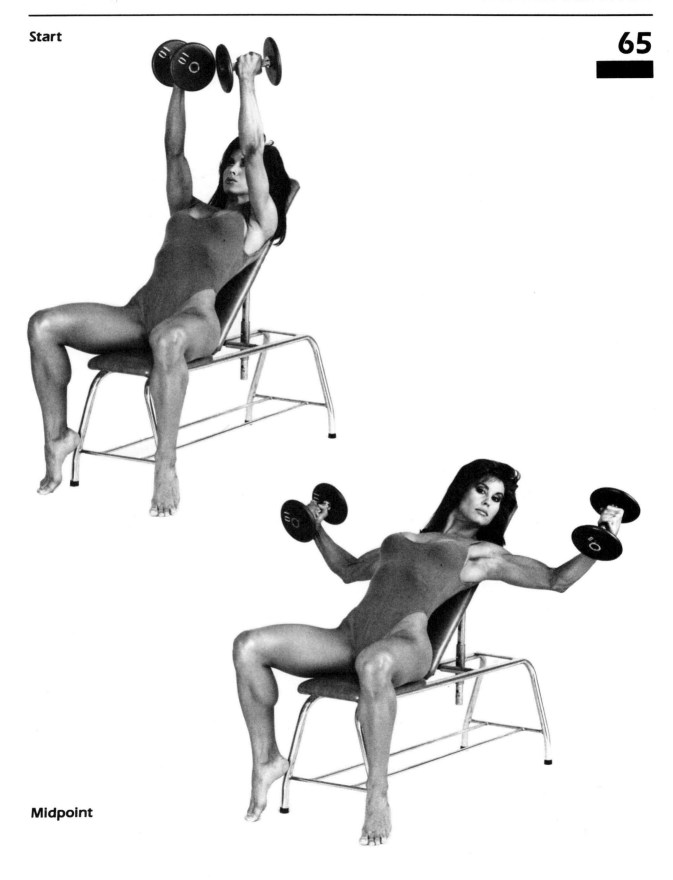

Midpoint

66

Start

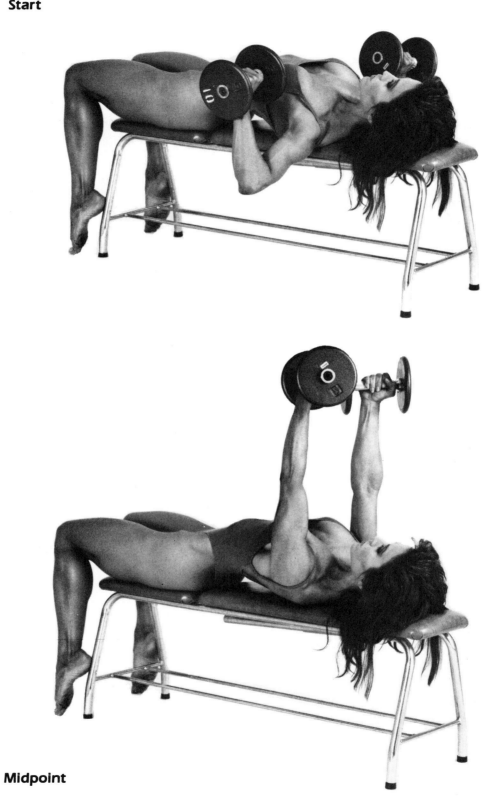

Midpoint

Flat Dumbbell Press

The flat dumbbell press perfects your entire chest area, especially the medial and outer pectorals. It uplifts sagging breasts. There is indirect stimulation of the frontal deltoids and the triceps.

POSITIONING

■ Lie on a standard flat exercise bench with a dumbbell in each hand and palms facing upward.

■ Place the dumbbells at each armpit, the disk of each dumbbell almost touching your armpit. You should feel a stretch in your chest and shoulders.

THE MOVEMENT

■ Raise the dumbbells, simultaneously rotating your wrists inward, until your arms are fully extended upward, with your palms facing behind you. Flex your pectoral muscles. (Rotating the wrists makes a "truer" contraction possible.)

■ Bending your elbows, lower the dumbbells until the plates graze your armpits. Stretch your pectorals, pushing your chest outward in order to get that full stretch.

■ Repeat the movement until you have completed your set.

REMEMBER

■ Be sure to extend your elbows downward and back on the down movement in order to get a full stretch in your chest.

■ Keep your mind on your pectoral muscles throughout the movement. Continually flex and stretch them.

■ Beware of the temptation to hold your breath. Breathe naturally or, better yet, exhale forcefully on the up motion and inhale deeply on the down motion.

68

Start

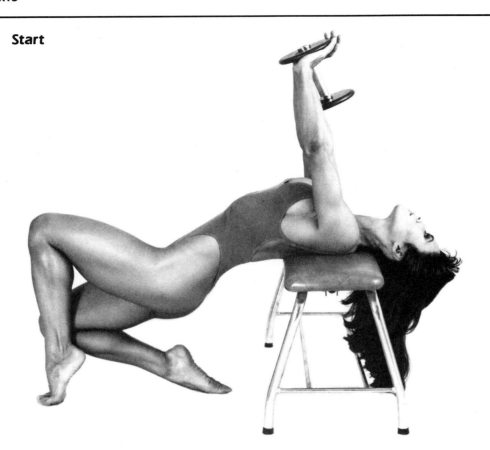

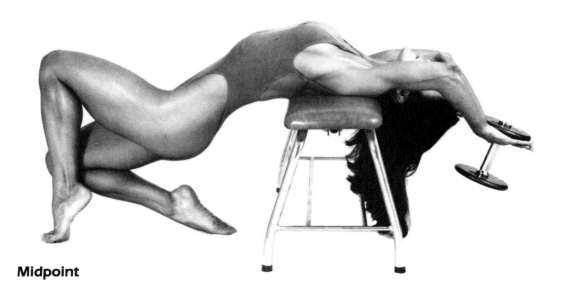

Midpoint

Cross-Bench Pullover

This exercise perfects the entire chest area. It stretches and expands the rib cage and indirectly affects the lats.

POSITIONING

■ Place a dumbbell beside you on a flat exercise bench and place your shoulders at the edge of the bench, letting your neck and head extend over the bench.

■ Grasp the dumbbell, with palms upward and thumbs crossed over, and hold the dumbbell at full arm's length above your chest area.

■ Place your feet a few inches apart and keep your hips down. Your legs and thighs should be in a near L position—your buttocks will be a bit lower. (I prefer to bend one leg because that keeps me low and enables me to stretch with a wider range of motion.)

THE MOVEMENT

■ Inhale with a deep breath as you lower the dumbbell behind you by bending your elbows slightly and extending your arms over and behind your head.

■ Lower the dumbbell until you feel a full stretch in your chest, keeping your buttocks down and arms close to your head.

■ Exhale and simultaneously flex (squeeze together) your pectoral muscles on the up motion to return to the start position. Flex again for a moment before you repeat the movement.

REMEMBER

■ Keep your energy focused on your pectoral (chest) muscles throughout the movement. Again, think of your arms as levers. Don't let your arms do the work. Continually stretch and flex your pectoral muscles.

■ Don't rush the movement. Maintain control and concentration for each repetition.

■ It takes time to get used to this exercise—it will seem awkward at first. Relax and enjoy the adjustment time. This is a soothing, calming exercise. You will eventually look forward to doing it.

70 Hand-on-Knee Isometric Contractions (Plus Variation)

These exercises develop the entire pectoral area, tightening, shaping, defining, and uplifting the pectoral muscles. You can do these anywhere.

POSITIONING

- Sit on the floor with your legs crossed.
- Place your right hand on your left knee, keeping your hand there throughout the exercise.
- Place your left fingertips on your right pectoral so that you can feel the contraction of your pectoral muscles as you perform the exercise.

THE MOVEMENT

- Focus on your knee as a solid base that provides the resistance as your arm, ever so slightly bent, fully extends and firmly presses it.
- Contract your right pectoral muscle for four to six seconds, using all the strength you have. When properly done, there will be a pleasing sensation of near pain.
- Relax for a second and repeat the movement five to eight times.
- Reverse your position and repeat the exercise for the left pectoral muscle.

REMEMBER

- To get the most effect on the upper pectoral muscle, shrug your shoulder upward slightly the last couple of seconds. Wow!
- To affect the lower pectoral more strongly, slope your shoulder downward as you flex and squeeze.
- Keep your mind riveted on your pectoral muscles throughout the movement. You are doing all the work here. There are no weights involved. Intensity of contraction is the key to results here.

TIP

To affect different areas of the chest, position your arms at different levels. To stimulate the upper pectorals more intensely, angle your arms at chin level (and for extra peak contraction, use the shrug technique here, too). To stimulate the medial and lower pecs, slope your shoulders downward as you lower the angle of your arms toward the floor.

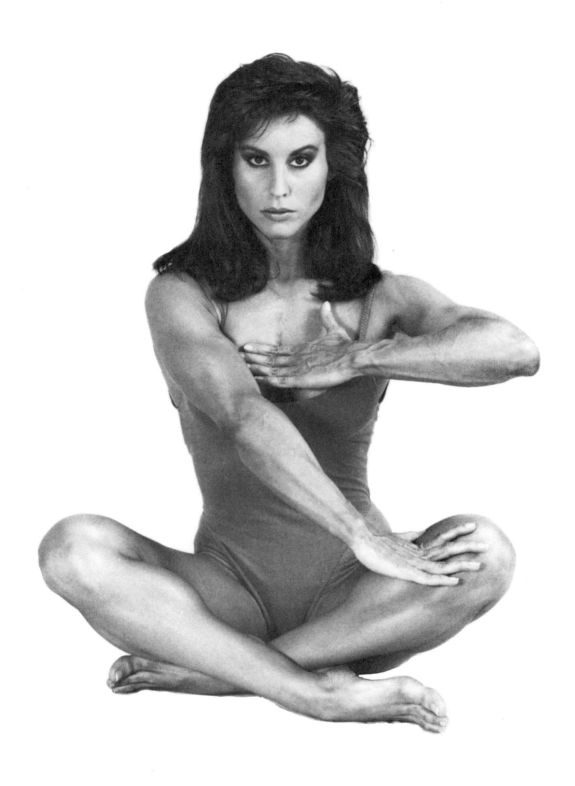

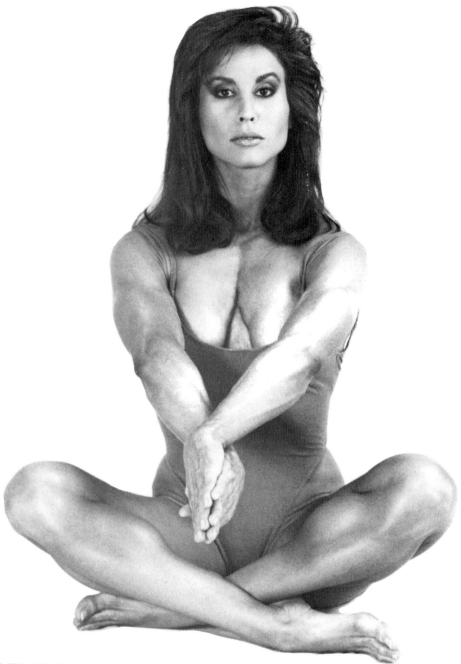

VARIATION

■ Seated in the same position, cross your forearms and clasp your hands, arms out in front of you and slightly bent.

■ Take a deep breath, then exhale as you straighten your arms and press the heels of your hands together, squeezing your chest muscles as hard as you can. Hold the contraction about four to six seconds. Repeat the movement five to eight times.

Flat Dumbbell Flye

This exercise perfects the entire pectoral chest area.

POSITIONING

■ Lie on your back on a flat exercise bench, holding a dumbbell in each hand. (The bench position is the only difference from the position assumed for the incline dumbbell flye. Refer to the photos for that exercise to check basics of the movement.)

■ Let your feet touch the floor comfortably on either side of the bench.

■ With palms facing each other, extend your arms straight up so that the dumbbells are in alignment with each other directly above your shoulder joints.

THE MOVEMENT

■ Slightly bend your arms and extend them downward in a semicircular movement until you feel a complete stretch in your upper pectoral (chest) area. Keeping your upper back flat against the bench, take a deep breath and push your chest slightly outward to get the full stretch.

■ Exhale forcefully as you bring the dumbbells back to start position and flex (squeeze together) your pectoral muscles.

■ Repeat the movement until you have completed your set.

REMEMBER

■ Keep your elbows slightly bent throughout the exercise.

■ Keep your mind on your pectoral muscles throughout the exercise.

■ Breathe naturally. Don't hold your breath.

■ Try to keep your arms on the same plane as your shoulders—in other words, keep your elbows back toward your head.

74 GYM CHEST ROUTINE

Incline Dumbbell Flye

Follow the instructions on page 64.

Pec Deck Flye

Pec deck flyes build up the entire pectoral area, especially the inner area. They help to develop the look of "cleavage."

POSITIONING

- Position yourself in the seat of the pec deck machine, adjusting the seat so that your upper arms are nearly parallel to the floor as you perform the exercise.
- Place your elbows behind the pads and grip the upper edge of the pads lightly. (Some machines have a specific place for your hands.)
- The machine will pull your elbows outward until you feel a complete stretch in your chest. You are ready to begin.

THE MOVEMENT

- Bring the pads together by exerting effort with your chest muscles. The pads should end up touching each other in the center of your chest. Flex (squeeze together) your pectoral muscles, and return to start position, letting the weights stretch your chest.
- Repeat the movement until you have completed your set.
- For different effects on your pecs, try adjusting the seat position higher or lower once you have mastered the movement in the usual position.

REMEMBER

- Don't jerk the pads in a desperate attempt to perform the exercise. If it's too heavy, lighten the weight. Perfect form is a must.
- Never let the pads return by themselves. *You* return them slowly to start in full control.
- Be careful to do the work with your pectoral muscles and not with your shoulders or arms. Keep your mind on your chest and your body stationary.
- Don't hold your breath. Breathe in as you stretch your chest and exhale as you exert your energy.

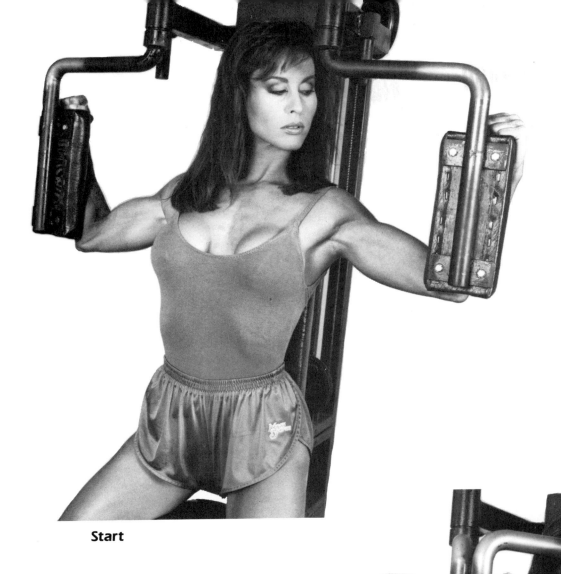

Start

Midpoint

Start

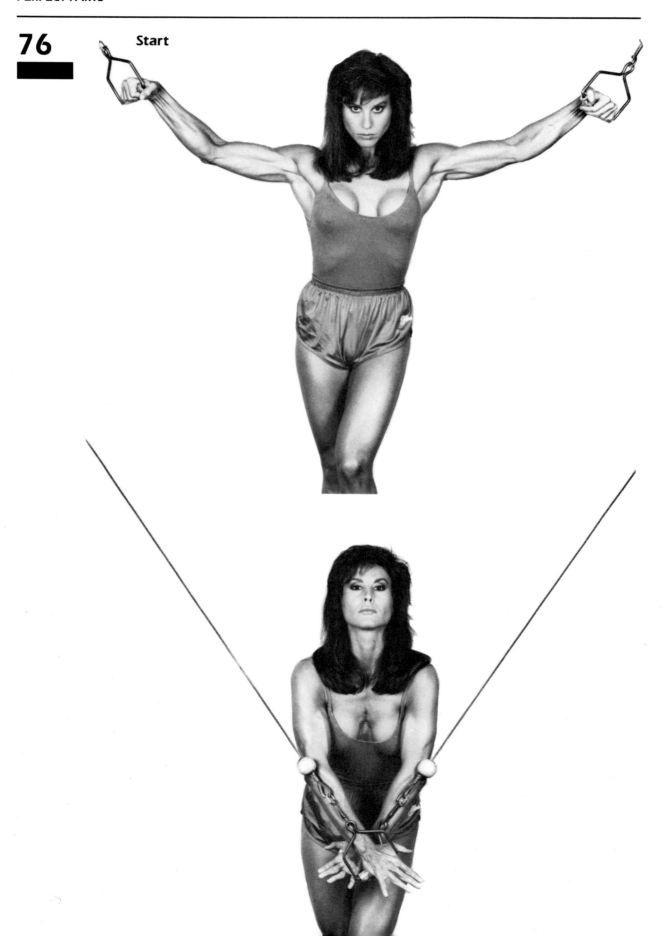

Cable Crossover

This exercise works to develop the entire chest area. It defines and lifts the pectoral muscle.

POSITIONING

■ Take hold of one handle of the crossover pulley device with each hand and stand in the center of the workout area. (This should be located in front of a mirror.) Keep your feet about shoulder width apart, or stand with one foot forward for better stability.

■ Raise your arms to a point where you feel a stretch in your chest. This is the point to which you will return after each rep.

■ The palms of your hands should be facing downward. You may bend forward slightly. Plant your feet firmly.

THE MOVEMENT

■ Flex your pectoral (chest) muscles as you pull both handles downward until they cross each other at the center of your body, wrist over wrist, lower forearms touching.

■ Return to start position while you remain in complete control of the weights.

■ Repeat the movement until you have completed your set.

REMEMBER

■ Keep your mind on your chest muscles at all times.

■ Work with your pectorals, not with your arms. (Notice that I am not even grasping the handles in the finish position, so as to isolate my chest.)

■ Flex (squeeze) your pectorals on the down movement and stretch them on the up movement.

■ Remain in control of the weights at all times. Never let them pull your arms upward, and don't jerk them downward.

Cross-Bench Pullover

Follow the instructions on page 69.

Flat Dumbbell Flye

Follow the instructions on page 73.

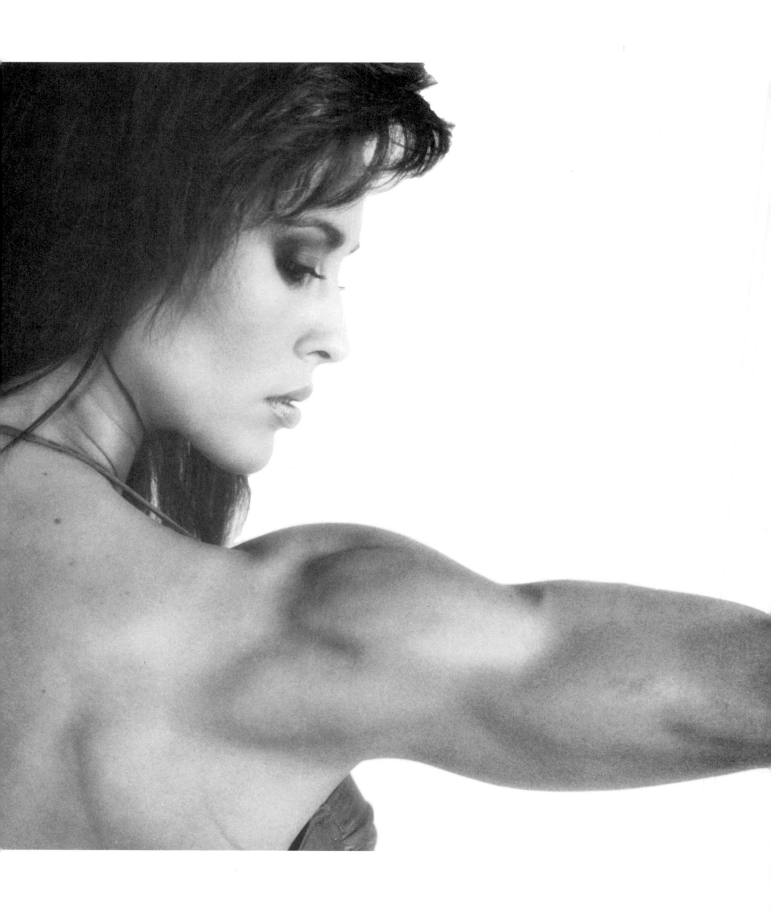

8

The Perfect Parts Shoulder Routine

The shoulders are a very sensual part of a woman's physique. Fashion designers have been well aware of this fact for decades and for this reason periodically place shoulder pads in women's clothing to create the look of the ever coveted hourglass figure. Well-shaped shoulders on a woman cause her to appear narrower at the waist. They also give her a youthful look and good posture.

Fortunately, you don't have to depend upon shoulder pads for "the look" or the posture. You can have it by working correctly with weights. Besides, you can't very well wear shoulder pads with a strapless gown or bathing suit. It's much better to have your own shapely shoulders.

Don't worry about getting "too big" in the shoulder area. Muscles don't happen that easily!

Every woman who has ever dreamed of wearing a strapless gown, swimsuit, or whatever but was insecure about her "bony" or fat, shapeless shoulders can achieve a perfectly balanced body and wear those clothes with confidence. Undeveloped shoulders give an unhealthy, weak appearance—a look of low self-esteem. Remember when your mom used to slap you on the back and say, "Straighten your shoulders"? Believe me, my shoulders used to be underdeveloped, too, before I started training with weights, and because of my underdeveloped shoulders, my thighs used to seem even bigger than they really were.

Down-sloping shoulders also make you appear tired and enervated—older.

Can you imagine how I would look if my shoulders were totally underdeveloped and the rest of my body were in the shape it is in now? See how one underdeveloped body part can destroy the overall appearance? I don't like pears, but I like resembling one even less. You can see why it is necessary to work on your shoulders in order to achieve a youthful, energetic, attractive look.

THE SHOULDER (DELTOID) MUSCLES

The deltoid muscles are located in the upper area of the shoulder. They consist of three "heads" that intertwine on the bone of the upper arm and collarbone. Your deltoids do the work of raising and rotating your arm. The anterior, or frontal, delts influence the movement in a forward direction, the posterior delts in a backward direction, and the medial head in a sideways direction.

Your deltoids should be equally developed in all three heads for perfectly balanced beauty. For this reason we have included exercises for each part of the muscle.

DEVELOPMENT

The deltoids are among the first muscles to show development on most women. You can expect to see something happening as early as three to six weeks, but you'll *feel* something immediately—after your first few workouts. They are relatively small muscles, and if you're not used to working them, they may be unusually sore for the first few weeks. Don't let that worry you. It's normal, and it's a good sign. It means that you are using muscles you have probably never used before, and you can expect to see quite a bit of progress in the near future.

When working your shoulders, don't forget to look in the mirror to check the progress of your rear deltoids. Well-developed rear deltoid muscles balance out large buttocks and make them appear smaller and in proportion.

Of all muscle groups, your deltoids are probably the most susceptible to overtraining. It is virtually impossible to perform any type of chest movement using dumbbells or barbell without stressing the frontal delts. Similarly, you cannot fully stimulate your back muscles to development without at the same time affecting your rear delts. Because of the combination effect, it's a good idea to exercise chest, shoulders, and back together in one workout session. (See the recommended combination routine indicated in chapter 5.)

EXERCISES

There are five exercises for a complete shoulder workout that works each head of the deltoids. Here is the list. (Home and gym shoulder routines are the same.)

HOME AND GYM SHOULDER ROUTINE

1. Standing side lateral
2. Seated alternating dumbbell press
3. Pee Wee lateral
4. Upright row
5. Seated bent-over lateral

Do seven to eleven repetitions for each of your three sets. If you find that you cannot get at least seven repetitions for your set, you have selected too heavy a weight. If you find that you're getting eleven repetitions too easily, you have selected too light a weight. Don't forget to raise your weight once it gets too easy (in about a month, I'd guess—everyone is different).

HOW OFTEN TO WORK OUT

See chapter 5 for details. If you are working only your shoulders or your shoulders and another body part or two, work out every other day or three times a week. If you have chosen to work your entire body and are following the four-day split routine, you will be working your shoulders twice a week. (Review page 47 for details on the whole-body split routine.)

WARM-UP/PRE-STRETCH

Stand with your feet in a natural position and your back erect. Extend your arms straight out to your sides, in line with your chest area. Rotate your arms backward in a circular motion to the count of ten, and then reverse the position and rotate them forward to the count of ten.

Now clasp your hands together behind your lower back and slowly straighten your arms. Feel the stretch in your shoulder joints. Hold there for a count of five. Then repeat. (This is the same stretch you did for your chest.) Keeping your hands clasped, bend your arms a little and rotate your shoulders forward ten times, then backward ten times. Again, repeat these movement immediately after completing your shoulder workout.

Before each exercise, do a set of fifteen to twenty repetitions at a very light weight. (You have to do this to warm up each deltoid head in turn.) This does not count as a set. Then you may begin your set, using an increased weight, of course.

82

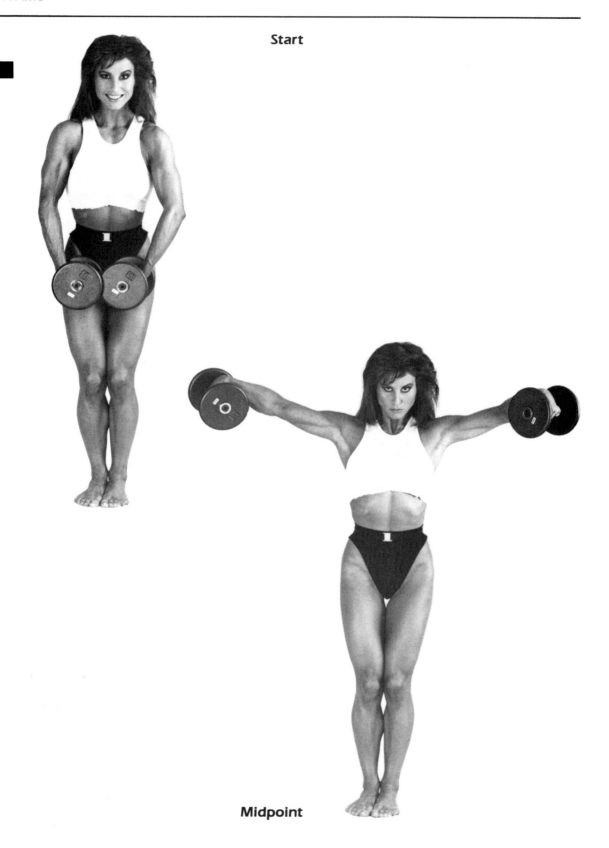

Midpoint

SHOULDER ROUTINE

Standing Side Lateral

This exercise perfects the medial (side) shoulder (deltoid) muscle. This movement will give nice width to your shoulders.

POSITIONING

- Grasp a light to moderate weight dumbbell in each hand, holding them with your palms facing each other.
- Lean forward just enough so that the dumbbells will be directly in front of your legs at the start of each repetition.

THE MOVEMENT

- Raise the dumbbells outward, leading with your outer wrists and elbows, until they are slightly higher than shoulder height. Your elbows will be slightly bent.
- Slowly return to start position and repeat the movement until you have completed your set.

REMEMBER

- Beware of the temptation to rock forward and to swing the dumbbells to the up position. This is a difficult but very effective isolation exercise, and it will be tempting to cheat. Instead of cheating, use a low weight at first (even as light as 3 pounds if necessary) and do the exercise *in perfect form*. There is plenty of time to raise your weights as you become more proficient at the exercise.
- Never let the dumbbells drop down to the start position. The down movement is as much a part of the exercise as the up movement.
- Keep your mind on your side deltoids throughout the exercise.

VARIATION

- You can also do this exercise while seated. It is more difficult, but you will get results faster. But first master the movement in a standing position; wait a few months before trying it in the seated position.

84

Start

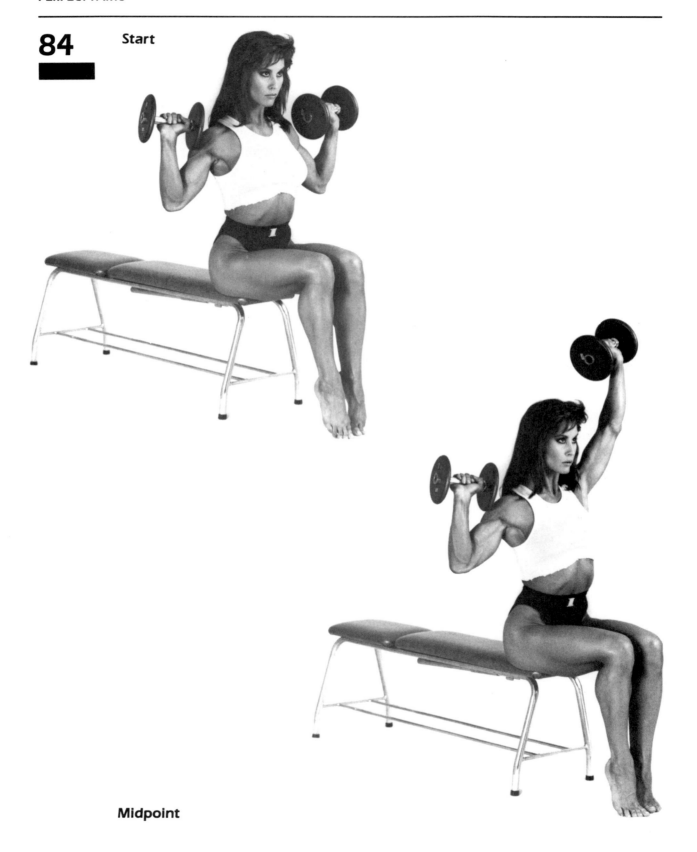

Midpoint

Seated Alternating Dumbbell Press

This exercise perfects the entire deltoid (shoulder) area, especially the front deltoid. It also indirectly stresses the triceps and trapezius muscles.

POSITIONING

- Sit at the edge of a flat exercise bench, facing a mirror if possible, while holding a dumbbell in each hand.
- Place your feet a comfortable width apart and sit with your back erect, looking directly ahead in the mirror.
- Hold the dumbbells at shoulder height, palms facing forward.

THE MOVEMENT

- Extend your right arm upward until it is fully extended.
- Bring your right arm back. When it is almost returned to start position, begin to extend your left arm. When it is fully extended your right arm should be back to start position.
- Bring your left arm back and extend the right arm up again in the same manner.
- Continue this alternating movement until you have completed your set.

REMEMBER

- Beware of the tendency to lean forward. Maintain an erect position throughout the movement.
- Be careful not to rock from side to side. Concentrate on maintaining your posture so that your shoulders do all the work.
- Feel the flex in your deltoid muscles on both the up and down movement as you maintain control of the weight.

86 Pee Wee Lateral

This exercise develops both the rear and medial deltoid muscles. The inspiration for it comes from Pee Wee Herman (who should definitely do a regular set or two for the rest of his life).

POSITIONING

■ Grasp a dumbbell in each hand and stand with your feet somewhat less than shoulder width apart and your hips thrust forward.
■ Holding the dumbbells with the outside of your wrists facing each other, move your hands behind you until the dumbbells nearly touch each other at about the center of your back.

THE MOVEMENT

■ Extend the dumbbells outward and upward in an arclike movement, leading with your outer wrists and elbows, until the dumbbells are shoulder height.
■ Slowly return to start position and feel the stretch in your shoulders.
■ Repeat the movement until you have completed your set.

REMEMBER

■ Keep your mind on your rear deltoid (shoulder) muscles throughout the movement.
■ Keep your hips thrust forward.
■ Don't yield to the temptation to swing the dumbbells into position. Keep a steady control on them as you raise and lower them deliberately for each repetition. Never let them simply drop to start position.
■ Don't allow your hips to sway back and forth in an effort to give yourself momentum and to relieve the shoulders of some of the work.

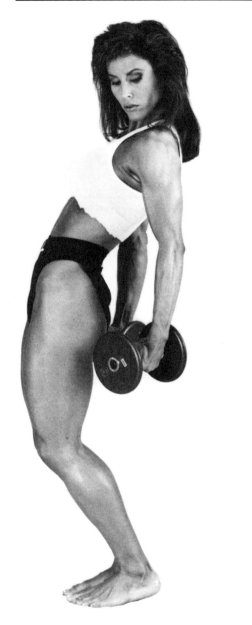

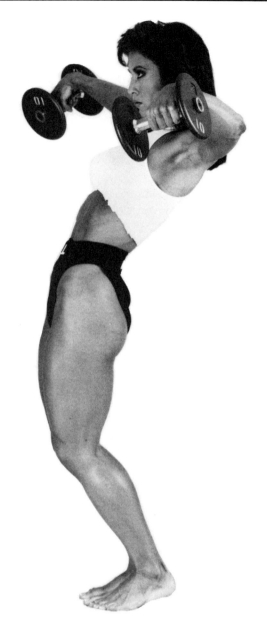

Start   **Midpoint**

88 Upright Row

The upright row develops the entire deltoid (shoulder) area as well as the trapezius muscles and indirectly stresses the biceps.

POSITIONING

■ Grasp a barbell, with your palms facing you. Place your hands about six to eight inches apart. (A wider grip can be used to stress the medial delts more.)
■ Stand with your feet a comfortable width apart and your body erect. Look in the mirror. Let the barbell rest against your upper thighs, with your arms fully extended downward.

THE MOVEMENT

■ Raise the barbell until it reaches your upper chest area or until it nearly grazes your chin, flexing your deltoids throughout the movement. Do not lean forward, and lift the barbell away from your body until it reaches your upper chest.
■ Return to the start position, keeping control of the barbell, and repeat the movement until you have completed your set.

REMEMBER

■ Never swing the barbell up. Be careful to control the barbell on the upward movement.
■ Resist the temptation to let the barbell simply drop to the start position.
■ Do not rock to and fro. Keep a steady erect stance.

Start

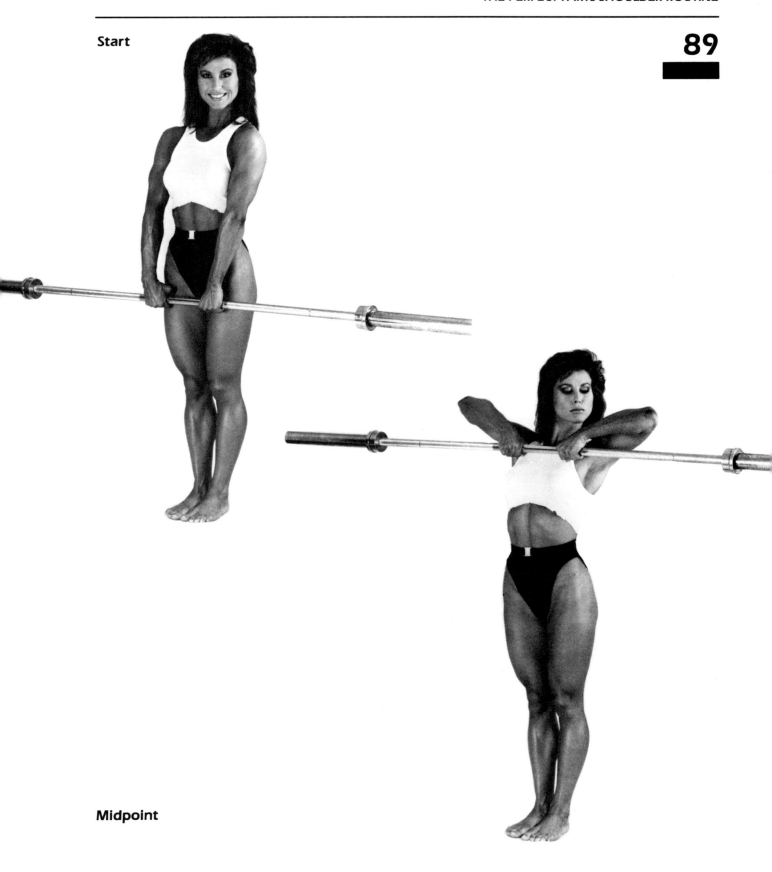

Midpoint

90

Start

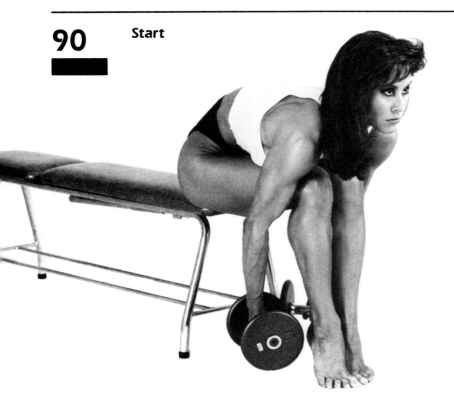

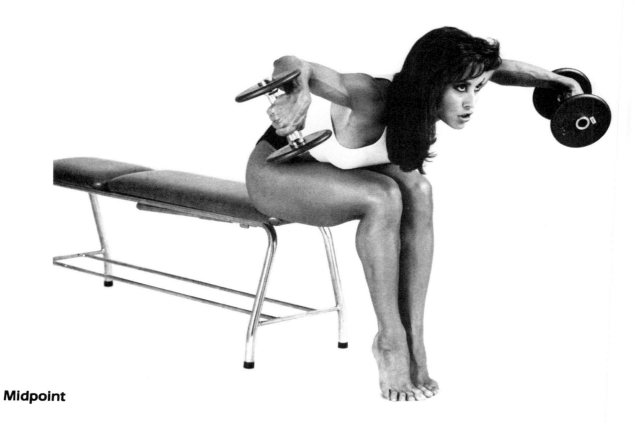

Midpoint

Seated Bent-Over Lateral

This exercise perfects the rear and side deltoid muscles.

POSITIONING

■ Sit at the edge of a flat exercise bench with a dumbbell held in each hand, palms facing each other.

■ Lean forward until your torso is nearly parallel to the floor and hold the dumbbells under your bent knees. The dumbbells should almost touch each other.

THE MOVEMENT

■ Extend your arms outward in an arclike movement. Your elbows should be slightly bent.

■ Raise the dumbbells until they are shoulder height, leading again with outer wrists and elbows and directing the movement of your shoulders forward toward your ears. This keeps the stress directly on the rear deltoids rather than on your lats.

■ Return to start position and feel the stretch in your shoulders.

■ Repeat the movement until you have completed your set.

REMEMBER

■ Resist the temptation to rise up to a sitting position. Keep your torso lowered and almost touching your knees at all times.

■ Don't swing the dumbbells up and never let them simply drop to the start position.

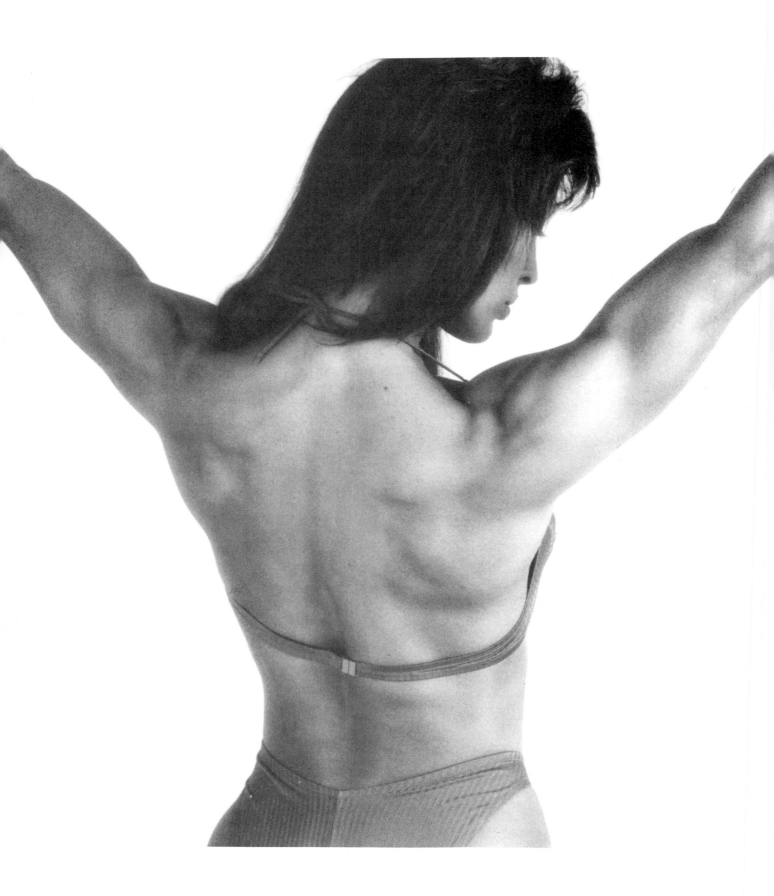

9

The _Perfect Parts_ Back Routine

The back contributes perhaps more to the overall shape of feminine physique than any other body part. Among other things, a statuesque, well-defined, V-shaped back gives a woman a smaller looking waist. Besides that, your back development determines your posture, because it is the latissimus dorsi (or "lat") muscles of the back that keep your shoulders from slumping. With good lat development, you will have a youthful, erect posture. Without it, you'll appear round-shouldered, tired looking, and yes, a good deal older.

It is the added width in your upper back when your latissimus dorsi are developed that makes your waist appear smaller, creating that athletic V shape. But I'm not talking about developing a bodybuilder's physique or the back of a wrestler. I'm talking about a toned, supple quality that breathes vigor. Naturally you'll look better in a backless summer dress or swimsuit, but even your winter clothes will drape more attractively on your figure. All it takes is enough development to provide lift to your shoulders. Suddenly your hips will appear to be narrower, and even your buttocks will appear smaller. It's like working as an artist, balancing body proportions to create an overall look. Bodybuilders, models, actresses, and others dependent on their looks for a living have done it for years.

Very few women use their back muscles to the point where they are sufficiently developed. Modern living does not require us to put our backs into physical activity to any great degree. While we can justifiably be glad that we don't have to do physical labor any more just to survive, we do pay a price for our comparatively luxurious way of

93

living—the lack of overall tone, strength, and symmetry we would otherwise have. Fortunately, the problem is relatively easy to correct.

Every woman should work on her back. Luckily, working on the back is not a tedious chore. On the contrary, it's rather enjoyable. In all the years of my working with women, I've never heard one of them complain, "I can't stand to work my back," although I've heard many complaints about exercising other body parts. I think it's because lots of tension regularly builds up in the neck and back over the course of the day. Before long the back is begging to be stimulated, and when it is, you are *so* relieved. In addition, the back is naturally strong and responds quickly to workouts.

THE BACK MUSCLES

The latissimus dorsi, or "lats," are the most prominent back muscles and originate from the spinal column near the middle of the back and the tailbone. They run upward and sideways and taper into the shoulder area, narrowing as they go. (They give the back its V shape.) The lats do the work of arching the shoulders, pulling the shoulders back and downward, and they also pull the arm back.

There are many other back muscles that enhance the beauty of a woman's back when developed. These include the rhomboids, the teres major and minor, supraspinatus, infraspinatus, thoracolumbar fascia and external oblique muscles. All of these muscles are strengthened and developed with the home or gym back routine given here. They work in combination to help pull and rotate the shoulders and arms. (There are only a couple of machine exercises that isolate the lats. Most back exercises work several muscles in the back as well as muscles in the arms.) The result of your working your back will not only be added beauty, it will be added strength in lifting and doing physical work in general, better posture, and a positive release of the tension that builds up in this area.

DEVELOPMENT

The back, especially the latissimus dorsi, develops slower than most other body parts. You will see some development of the smaller muscles of your back within three months, but it may take longer before you notice lat development. You will notice one thing much sooner: In about three weeks there will be an immediate improvement in your posture. Your shoulders will be less rounded, and you'll find you sit and walk with your head up. The process of development will have begun to make a noticeable difference, even though you may not see more muscle yet.

Don't be concerned about how long it takes to develop your lats to the point where you can see them becoming more defined. Let nature take its course. Everyone is different. Meanwhile, enjoy your new body awareness, and remember that once your lats are perfectly developed, they are yours for life, so it's worth the wait.

EXERCISES

There are five exercises for your back workout. If you are working at home, follow the home routine, which is given first. If you are working in a gym or fitness center, follow the gym routine, given toward the end of the chapter.

HOME BACK ROUTINE

1. One-arm dumbbell bent row
2. Barbell bent row
3. Deadlift
4. Seated dumbbell back lateral
5. Straight-arm body pull

GYM BACK ROUTINE

1. Lat pull-down to the rear
2. Lat pull-down to the front
3. Pulley row
4. Barbell bent row
5. One-arm dumbbell row

Do seven to eleven repetitions of each of your three sets. If you find yourself able to do more than eleven repetitions, it is time to raise your weight. Repeat the pre-stretch movement at the end of your back routine.

HOW OFTEN TO WORK OUT

You can work your back twice a week, but be sure to leave a day or two in between workouts. If you wish, you can work your back three times a week or every other day, but two times a week will be sufficient.

WARM-UP/PRE-STRETCH

Grab onto anything overhead that will safely support you in a hanging position with both feet off the ground, your arms fully extended above you. Hang for about fifteen seconds. Let your back stretch completely out. (If you are working out in the gym, you can use the lat pull-down bar by placing the pin on a heavy weight so that your body will be supported as you hang.)

Follow with a light set of fifteen to twenty repetitions for the first exercise before you do your regular three sets, and do a light warm-up set before each subsequent exercise. (This light set does not count as a full exercise set.)

96

Start

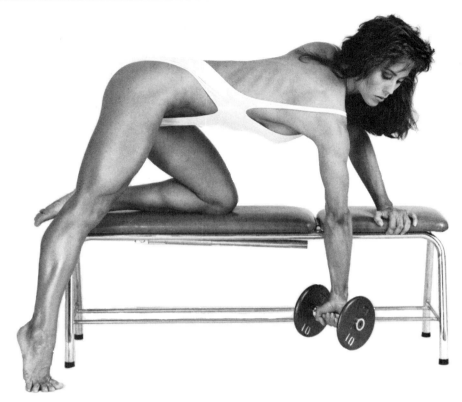

Midpoint

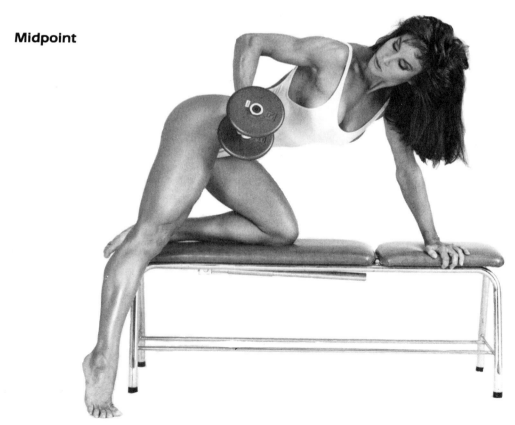

HOME BACK ROUTINE

One-Arm Dumbbell Bent Row

This exercise works to perfect the latissimus dorsi and the trapezius while indirectly stimulating the biceps.

POSITIONING

- Lean over a flat exercise bench, placing your right knee and right hand on the bench for support.
- Place your left foot firmly on the floor and keep it there throughout the exercise.
- Hold a dumbbell in your left hand, palm toward your body and elbow away from your body, and let the dumbbell pull your arm straight down. You will feel a stretch in your left back muscles. Your arm should be perpendicular to the floor.

THE MOVEMENT

- Raise the dumbbell by pulling your arm up, simultaneously rotating your arm slightly as you aim your outer wrist toward your hip.
- Aim your elbows as high as possible so you feel the flex in your back muscles.
- Control the weight as you return to start position and feel the dumbbell stretch the left of your back. Let the dumbbell hang in your hand for a second before repeating the movement.
- Repeat the movement until you have completed your set.
- Repeat the set for your other arm.

REMEMBER

- Do the movement slowly and deliberately. If you do it too quickly, momentum will rob you of the precious muscle contraction you should be aiming for.
- Keep your mind on your working back muscles throughout the exercise, and make sure that your back and *not* your arms or shoulders are doing the work.
- Do not rest between arms. You have a natural rest period for one arm while the other is working.

98

Start

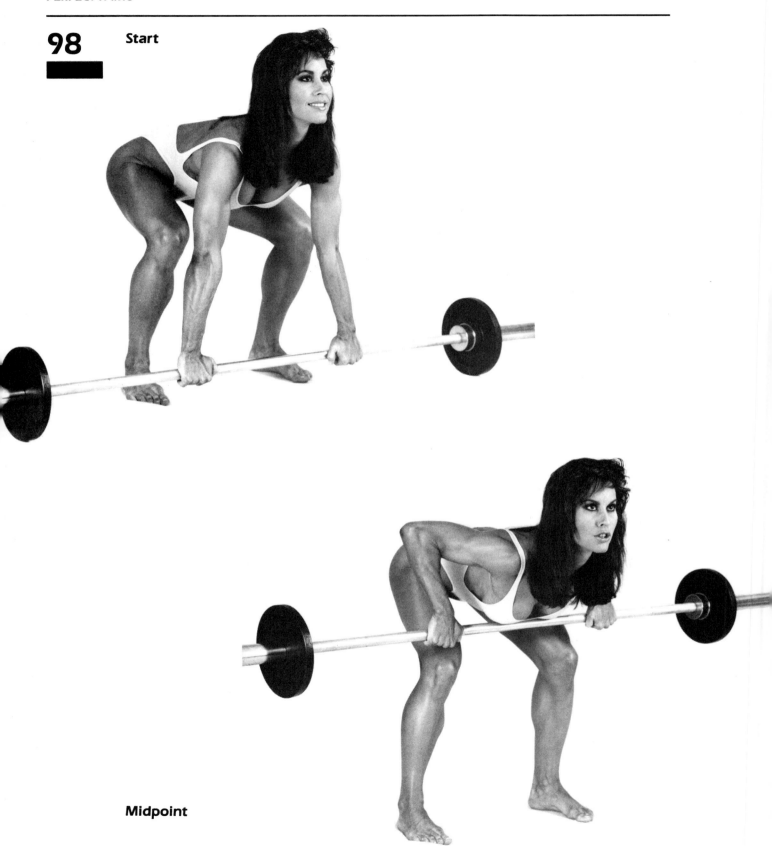

Midpoint

Barbell Bent Row

In addition to perfecting the latissimus dorsi, trapezius, and erector spinae, this exercise helps develop the biceps and indirectly stimulates the rear deltoids and the forearms.

POSITIONING

■ Place a barbell on the floor in front of you and position your feet about four inches wider than shoulder width apart.

■ Bend at the knees and, with your back arched, grip the barbell, palms facing your body, and hands a bit more than shoulder width apart.

■ Let your arms hang down straight to the floor as you allow the weight of the barbell to stretch your back muscles.

■ Bend over until your torso is parallel to the floor, holding your back arched to ensure proper contraction of the muscles there.

THE MOVEMENT

■ Pull the barbell up until it barely touches your rib cage, keeping your elbows close to your body throughout the exercise and your back arched so that you feel the flex in the back muscles.

■ Return to start position in full control, letting the barbell stretch out your back muscles as you reach the lowest point of the down movement.

■ Repeat the movement until you have completed your set.

REMEMBER

■ Raise the barbell slowly while mentally concentrating on your latissimus dorsi muscles. Never jerk the barbell up.

■ Never let the barbell simply drop to the down position. Realize that the down movement is half the exercise. Slowly lower the barbell in full control.

■ Be sure that your arms are fully extended before you begin each new rep. This will ensure a full stretch in your back muscles and lead to better results.

100 Deadlift

With deadlifts you perfect both the lower back muscles, particularly the erector spinae, and the upper back muscles. You also indirectly stimulate the muscles of the forearms, the thigh, and the buttocks.

POSITIONING

■ Step up to a barbell and stand with your feet shoulder width apart.
■ Arch your back and keep it arched and contracted as you bend at the knees to grasp the barbell. The palms of your hands should be facing you and positioned shoulder width apart on the bar.

THE MOVEMENT

■ Keeping your back arched and your buttocks tight, lift the barbell by straightening your legs. The barbell should be resting against your thighs in the finish position.
■ Lower the weight by bending your knees again, keeping your back tightly contracted.

REMEMBER

■ Do the movement slowly.
■ Concentrate on your lower back and buttocks throughout the exercise. Tell your lower back to be strong and your buttocks to help out.

Start

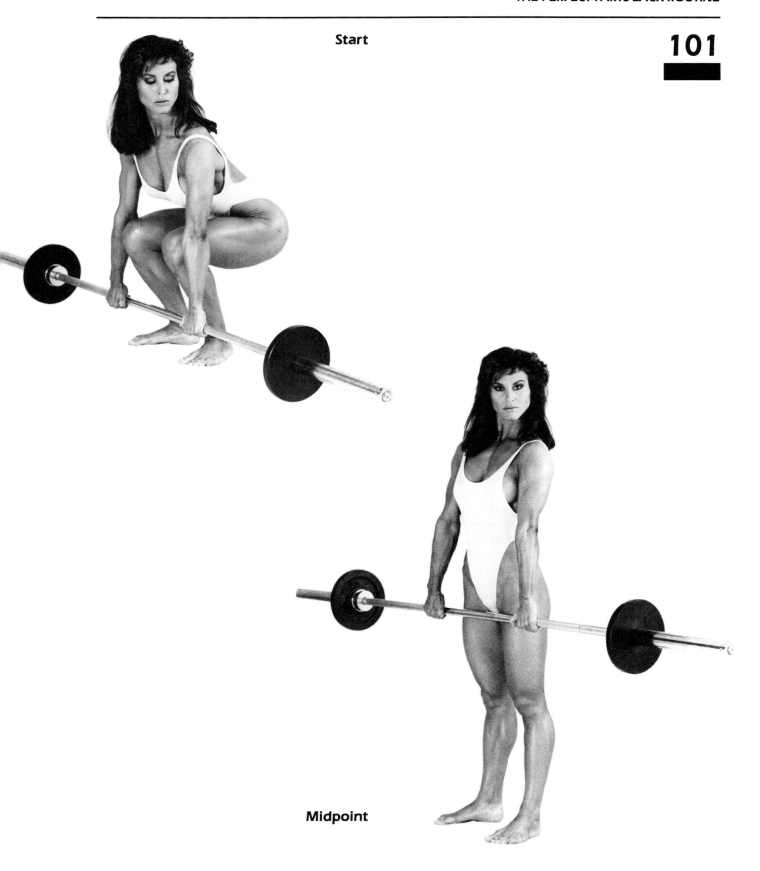

Midpoint

102

Start

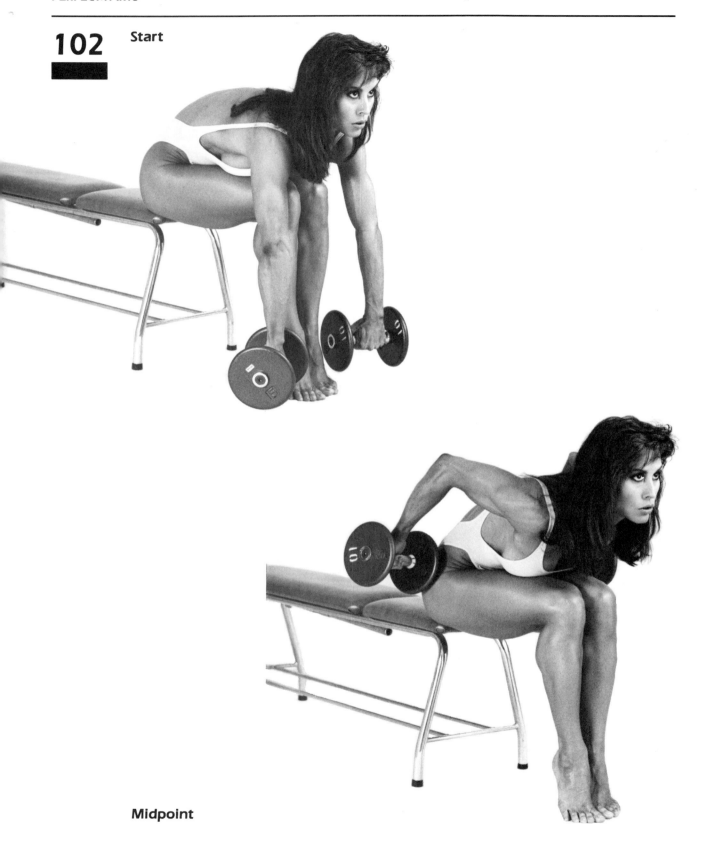

Midpoint

Seated Dumbbell Back Laterals

103

This exercise perfects the upper back and trapezius muscles.

POSITIONING

- Sit at the edge of a flat exercise bench and lean forward as far as you can.
- Hold a dumbbell in each hand, with your palms facing behind you.
- Position the dumbbells so that they are close together by your feet, as shown in the photograph.

THE MOVEMENT

- Raise your arms up and back, bringing the dumbbells to hip level. (Your hands will rotate so that palms face forward.) Keep your elbows close to your sides and as high as possible.
- While doing this, flex (squeeze together) your shoulders as if you were trying to grip something with the center of your back.
- Return to start position and let your upper back stretch completely as you rotate your hands so that your palms face behind you again.
- Repeat the movement until you have completed your set.

REMEMBER

- Don't get this exercise mixed up with seated rear laterals, a shoulder exercise where you lean forward and extend your arms out from your sides widely and forward to work your rear deltoid (shoulder) muscles more directly. In *this* exercise you must keep your elbows close to your sides and behind you at all times.
- Flex your upper back muscles continually on the up movement.
- Lower the weight slowly. Don't just let it drop back to the down position.
- Strive for a full stretch at the bottom of the movement.

104 Straight-Arm Body Pull

The straight-arm body pull works to develop the latissimus dorsi (lats) and the lower back (notably the erector spinae).

POSITIONING

- Stand two feet away from a sturdy chair back. Place the palms of your hands close together, flat on the edge of the chair back.
- Bend your knees, arch your back, and thrust your buttocks area out. Keep the heels of your feet flat on the ground.
- Your arms should be extended so that you feel a stretch in the lat area.

THE MOVEMENT

- With nothing but lat strength, pull in toward the chair. Your elbows will go inward, close to your body as you flex your lats and shoulder blades back and downward.
- As you pull in, rock forward on the balls of your feet and straighten your body at the hips.
- Feel the tension in your latissimus dorsi area as you flex your lat muscles and the middle of your back as hard as possible, and hold the flex for a couple of seconds.
- Return to start to stretch your lats fully and repeat the movement until you have completed your set.

REMEMBER

- It would be very easy to pull in and out without using tension, but then absolutely nothing would happen as a result of your effort.
- You *must* concentrate through every moment of this exercise. Keep your mind on your latissimus dorsi muscles and flex hard on the pulling movement.
- Your lats should be doing the work. Use your arms only to position yourself properly; do not use them to perform any of the work.

Start

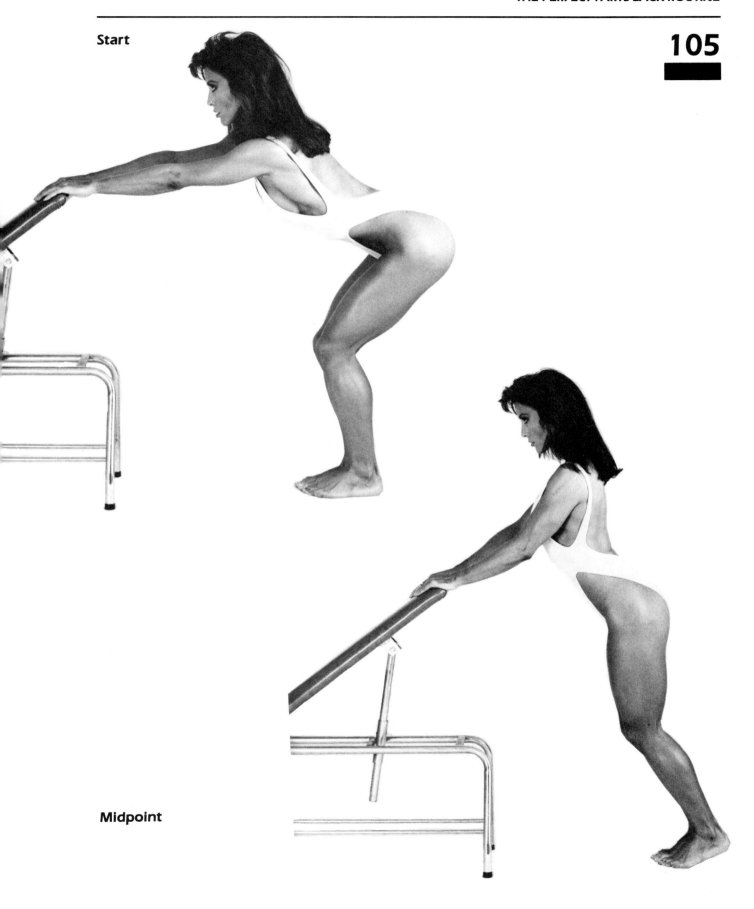

Midpoint

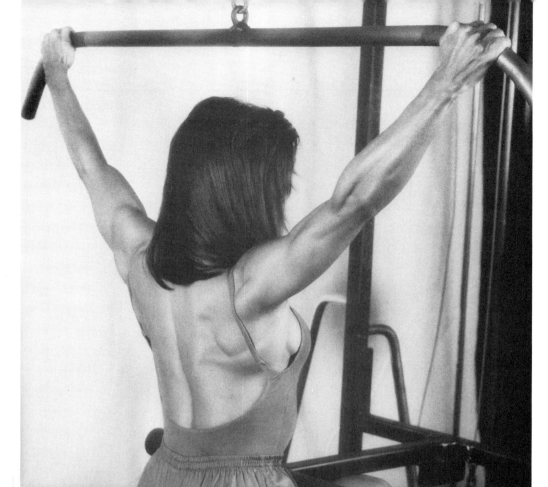

Start

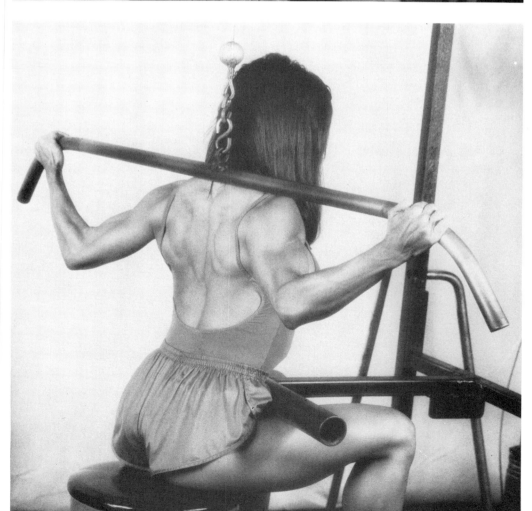

Midpoint

GYM BACK ROUTINE

Lat Pull-down to the Rear

This exercise perfects the latissimus dorsi and indirectly stimulates the biceps and forearm.

POSITIONING

■ Grasp the handles of the lat pull-down bar six inches wider than shoulder width, palms away from you. Let the weights stretch out your back as you fully extend your arms upward.
■ Place yourself in position on the seat, your knees held firmly under the restraining bar.

THE MOVEMENT

■ Arch your back to keep it tight and contracted as you pull the bar downward until it touches your trapezius muscles. Do the work with your lats. Think of your arms as assistants only. (You may lean forward *slightly* to get the bar in the proper finish position.)
■ Maintaining full control, return to start position and let the weights stretch your back.
■ Repeat the movement until you have completed your set.

REMEMBER

■ Avoid the temptation to jerk the weight downward and let it pull and control *you* on the way up. Instead control the weight on both up and down movements for each repetition of your set. Picture the nice hourglass V shape you'll have.
■ Flex (squeeze) your lats on the way down each time.
■ Beware of the temptation to let your body rise from the seat. Remain firmly seated as you work.

Start

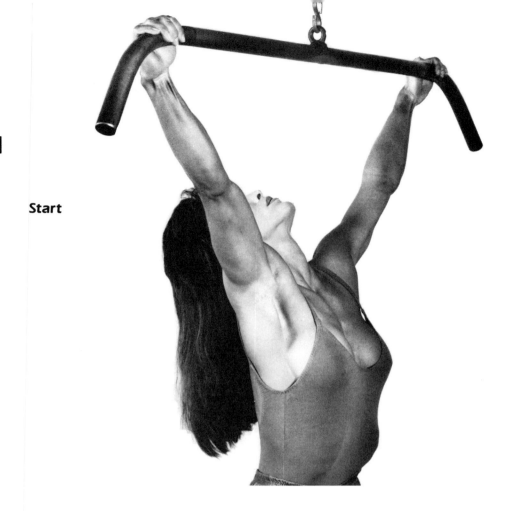

Midpoint

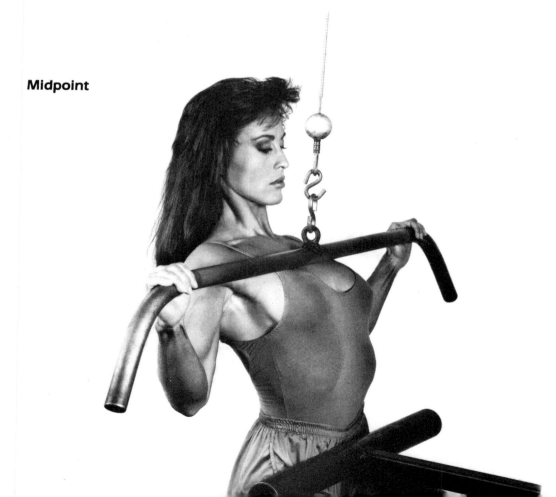

Lat Pull-down to the Front

109

These pull-downs also perfect the lats and indirectly stimulate the biceps and forearms.

POSITIONING

■ *Same as for lat pull-downs to the rear.*

THE MOVEMENT

■ Lean slightly back and pull the bar downward until it touches your upper chest. Keep your mind on your lat muscles the whole time.

■ Flex your lat muscles and return to start position.

■ Stretch your lats and repeat the movement until you have completed your set.

REMEMBER

■ You will be stronger in lat pull-downs to the front than in lat pull-downs to the rear.

■ Be sure to control the movement at all times.

■ Do the work with your back, not with your arms.

■ Do not rock your body backward. Instead, expand your chest upward to meet the bar as you pull it down.

110

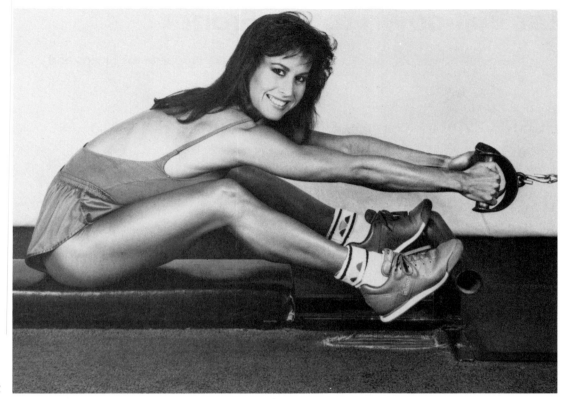

Start

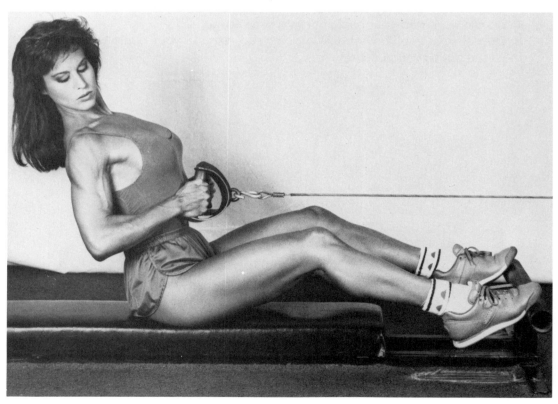

Midpoint

Pulley Row

Pulley rows perfect the entire back area, especially the trapezius, latissimus dorsi, and erector spinae. They indirectly stimulate the biceps, rear deltoids, and forearms.

POSITIONING

■ Sit in the seat of the pulley-row machine, holding the parallel-grip handles with palms facing each other.
■ Place your feet on the foot-rest bar and bend your knees slightly.
■ Extend your arms fully and lean forward to let the weights stretch your lats and lower back muscles fully.

THE MOVEMENT

■ Pull the handles toward your waist, keeping your body perpendicular to the floor. Arch your back at the same time. Avoid the temptation to bend backwards.
■ Touch the handles to your waist area.
■ Slowly return to start position, letting the weight stretch your back again.
■ Repeat the movement until you have completed your set.

REMEMBER

■ Don't jerk the weight toward your waist. Slowly pull it as you focus on your lat muscles.
■ Do not let your arms do most of the work.
■ Be careful not to lean way back on the pull-in position. Keep your body as straight as possible.
■ As you master control with your back muscles, strive for a rhythmic motion through each set while maintaining perfect form.

Barbell Bent Row

Follow the instructions on page 99.

One-Arm Dumbbell Bent Row

Follow the instructions on page 97.

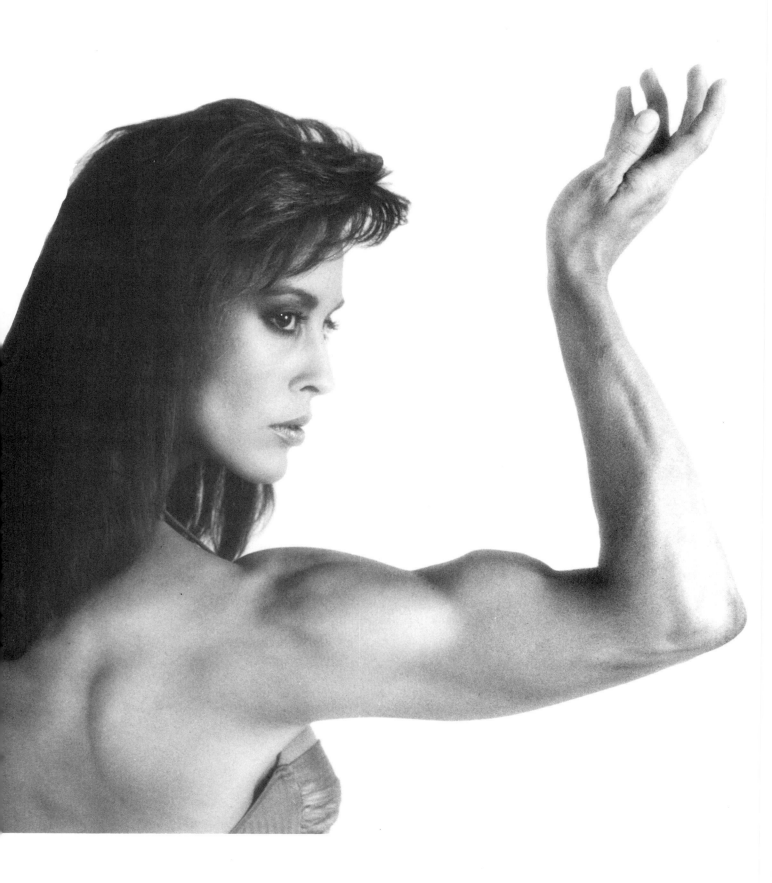

10

The **Perfect Parts** Biceps Routine

The biceps is the muscle that immediately comes to mind when you think of muscles. It comprises the forward side of the upper arm, balancing out the triceps muscle. Everyone knows how to flex a biceps. It's the one we show off when someone asks us to "make a muscle."

But the biceps is not just for showing off. It can add sensuality and balance to a woman's arm. A curvaceous, tightly formed biceps muscle is very attractive. Besides that, it gives you real strength in your arms.

Undeveloped biceps give the arm an unattractive sticklike appearance and draw attention to the hips and legs. An immediate comparison is made between the "skinny arms" and big hips (or legs, if you happen to have big legs).

If you are physically active, your biceps are probably somewhat developed already. You may be worrying, "Will I get too big?" Not with this routine. What you *will* get is a more shapely, fully formed biceps. Even if your biceps is already partially developed, it is probably not fully developed, because the normal body movements you do don't systematically force you to fully extend and contract your arm. The movement is haphazard, and the result is that the biceps is probably only partially developed, if it's developed at all.

As you know, muscular development happens only as a result of demands placed on a particular muscle or muscle group. So if there's no more stimulation than the usual day-to-day activities, you probably can't expect much in the way of development.

Curiously, some daily activities will contribute unexpectedly to muscle develop-

113

ment. When I was in my teens, I had long, heavy hair. I brushed it every day from the top of my scalp all the way to the ends, and I noticed a biceps muscle when I did so. Without actually intending to exercise my arm, I was moving it through a full range of movement and as a result experienced *some* development. Unfortunately, I never alternated hands when I brushed my hair, so the development I experienced was all on one side.

That's fairly typical of day-to-day routines. To the extent they do contribute to muscle development, it's generally limited and often uneven. Not until you consciously balance demands on your muscles in a regular workout routine will you find yourself developing the perfectly balanced body parts you long for.

THE BICEPS MUSCLE

The biceps is a two-headed muscle originating in the shoulder blade area and ending in the forearm. When developed, the two "bellies" of the muscle form a curve about halfway down the arm. The biceps works to bend or flex the arm at the elbow.

DEVELOPMENT

The biceps is a small muscle and is quickly stimulated, therefore three exercises are enough to achieve your goal. The triceps also needs only three exercises since it, too, is a small muscle. It is one of the first muscles to respond to the weights. You should see some development in about three to six weeks. The biceps is also easily "pumped up" (engorged with blood) after an intense workout. It stays pumped for about two hours, then returns to normal size. If you see this happen, take it as a sign that you have worked out especially hard that day.

EXERCISES

There are three exercises for the biceps in this routine. They are the same whether you are working out at home or in a gym or fitness center.

HOME AND GYM BICEPS ROUTINE

1. Standing alternate dumbbell curl
2. Angled simultaneous dumbbell curl (superset with the standing alternate dumbbell curl)
3. Standing barbell curl

Do three sets of seven to eleven repetitions for each exercise. If you find yourself able to do more than eleven repetitions, it is time to raise your weight.

HOW OFTEN TO WORK OUT

Work your biceps three times a week or every other day, unless you are working your entire body and following the split routine, in which case you will be working them twice a week.

WARM-UP/PRE-STRETCH

Sit on the floor, with legs and feet together. Position your arms straight down at your sides, with the palms of your hands flat on the floor, your fingers pointing behind you. Keeping your hands stationary, slowly scoot your body forward until you feel a pleasingly painful stretch in your biceps. (You will also feel a nice stretch in your shoulders.) Hold the stretch for a slow count of ten, then "walk" your hands up to your sides again and repeat the movement.

Follow this stretching movement with one set of fifteen to twenty repetitions of the standing alternate dumbbell curl using a light weight. Remember, this does not count as one of your regular three sets.

Repeat the stretch movement following completion of your biceps workout.

Start

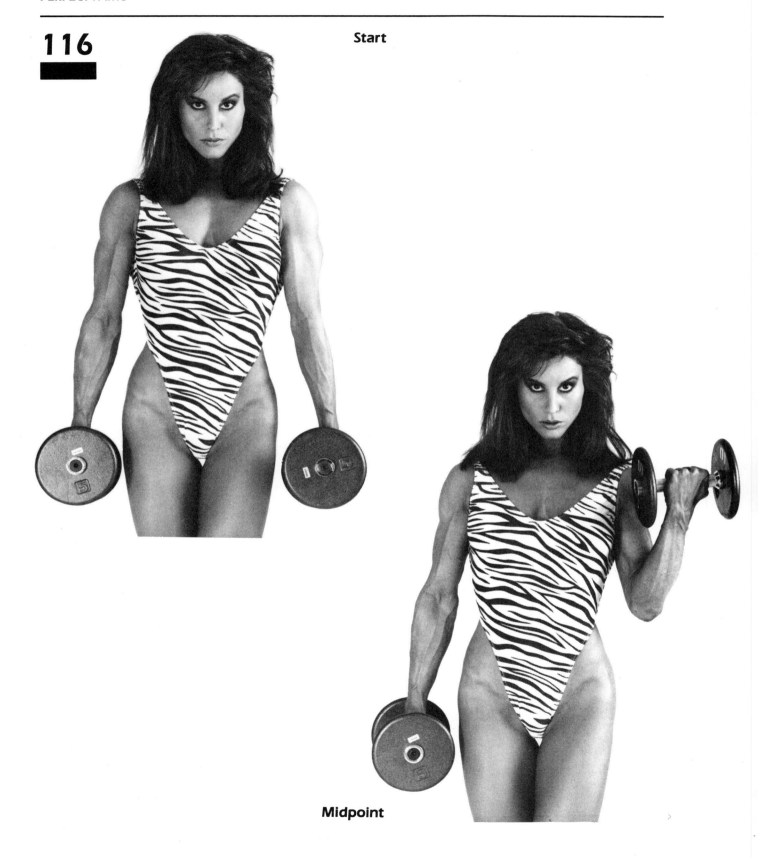

Midpoint

BICEPS ROUTINE

Standing Alternate Dumbbell Curl

The standing alternate dumbbell curl perfects the entire biceps muscle and the forearm. Superset the movement with the angled simultaneous seated dumbbell curl.

POSITIONING

- Stand in front of a mirror, with your feet a natural width apart.
- Grasp a dumbbell in each hand, with palms facing each other.
- Let your arms hang straight down at your sides. Keep your elbows close to your sides and your back erect throughout the exercise.

THE MOVEMENT

- Bend your left arm to curl the dumbbell up toward your left shoulder.
- As the dumbbell approaches your shoulder, rotate your wrist a quarter turn so that your palm faces up.
- As you complete the upward movement on the left, begin to curl the right dumbbell in the same way until it reaches your shoulder, meanwhile lowering the left dumbbell and rotating the left wrist back to the start position.
- Continue alternately to curl and lower your arms until you have completed your set.
- Flex (squeeze) the biceps muscle in either arm on the up movement and control the biceps muscle on the down movement until your arm is fully extended and you achieve a stretch.

REMEMBER

- Do not yield to the temptation to sway your body to help you finish a rep.
- Keep the movement strict and deliberate.
- Take no rest between movements when supersetting.

118

Start

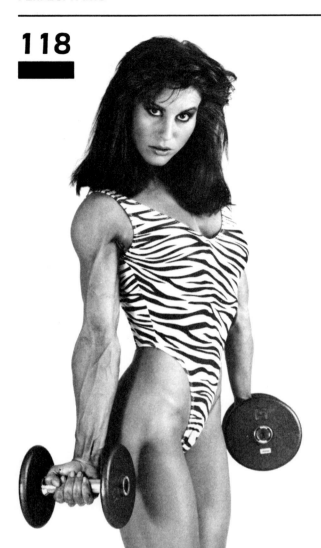

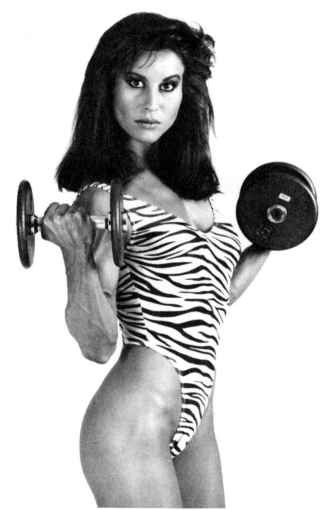

Midpoint

Angled Simultaneous Dumbbell Curl

119

This exercise also perfects the entire biceps muscle and the forearm.

POSITIONING

- Grasp a dumbbell in each hand, with your palms facing outward.
- Keep your back erect.
- Hold your elbows close to your sides throughout the exercise.
- Let your arms hang down at your sides and angle the dumbbells outward at an angle from your body.

THE MOVEMENT

- Raise the dumbbells simultaneously until they reach shoulder height and you cannot possibly curl any further.
- Flex your biceps muscles as you complete the movement, then slowly return to start position.
- Feel the stretch in your biceps muscles.
- Keep your elbows close to your sides and repeat the movement until you have completed your set.

REMEMBER

- Never let your elbows wander away from your sides.
- Keep the dumbbells angled outward.
- Don't start leaning forward and rocking back in an effort to take stress off the biceps. Perfect motion—that's the goal.

Start

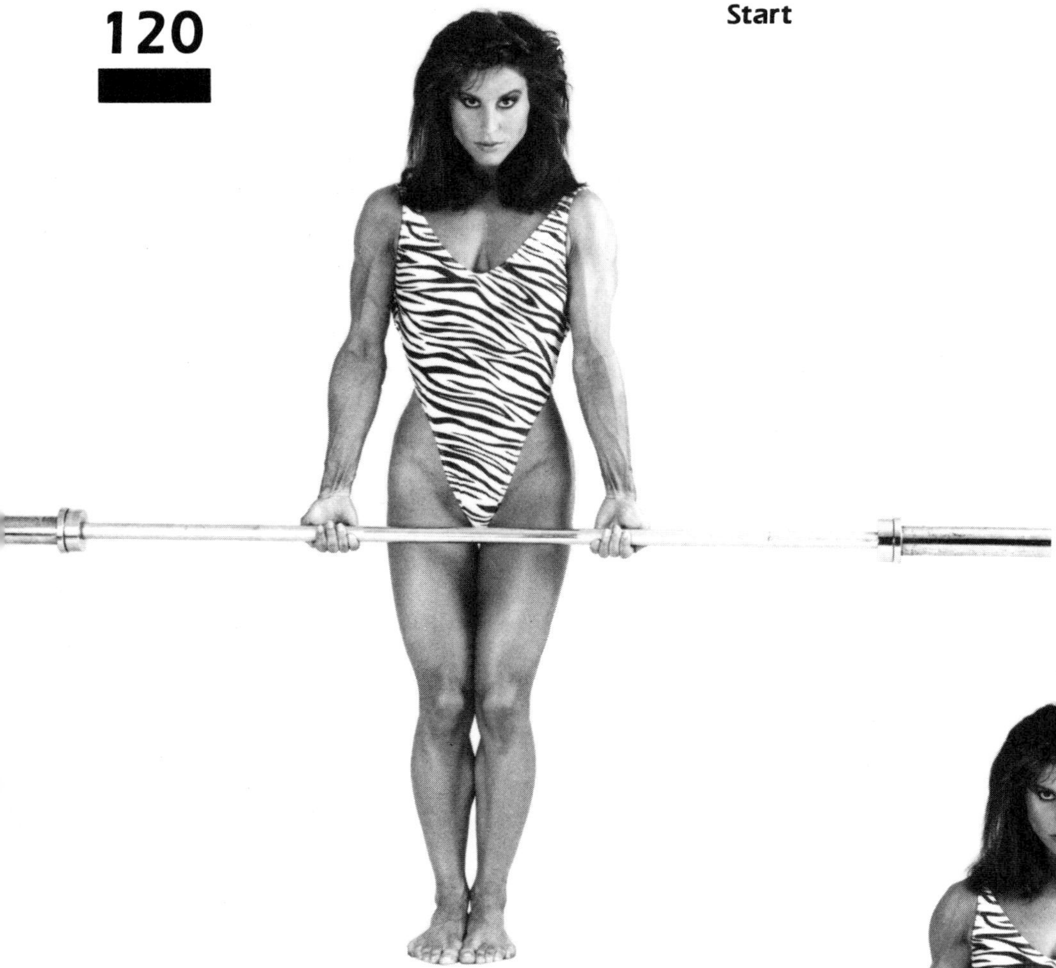

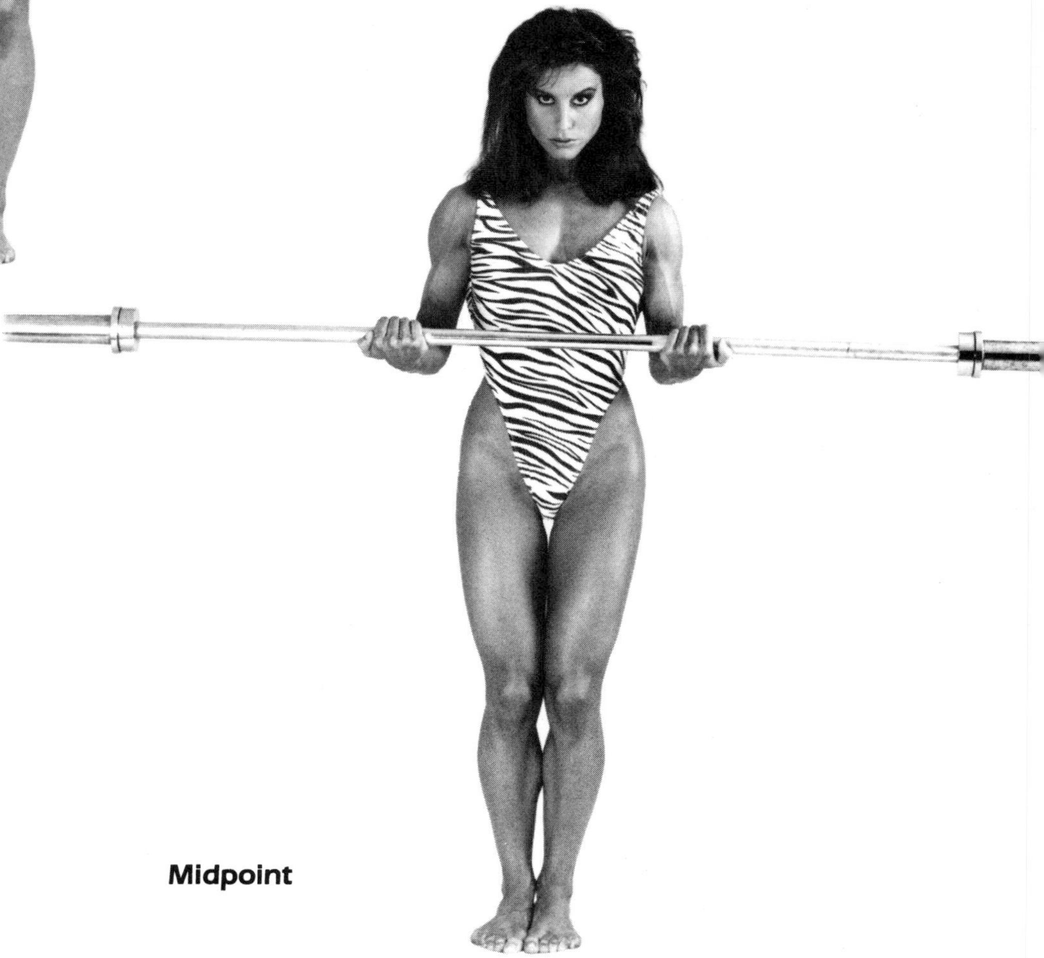

Midpoint

Standing Barbell Curl

121

This exercise perfects the entire biceps muscle.

POSITIONING

- Grasp a barbell with hands at shoulder width and palms facing outward. Let the barbell stretch your arms in a fully extended position.
- Keep your arms close to your sides but *slightly* in front of your body throughout the movement.
- Stand with your feet in a natural position.

THE MOVEMENT

- Flexing your biceps through the complete upward movement, raise the barbell to your upper body until it reaches the highest position, close to your shoulders.
- Return to start position in full control of the barbell and repeat the movement until you have completed your set. Be sure to let the barbell stretch your biceps fully on the down movement. *Feel the stretch.*

REMEMBER

- Lock your wrists and keep them locked throughout the movement.
- Maintain a fluid, controlled movement. Never jerk the barbell up, and always control it going down.
- Beware of the temptation to cheat by rocking back and forth in an effort to give yourself momentum and thus avoid pushing the barbell solely with biceps strength. Remember, the whole idea is to stimulate this muscle to peak contraction. Get the most out of your efforts.

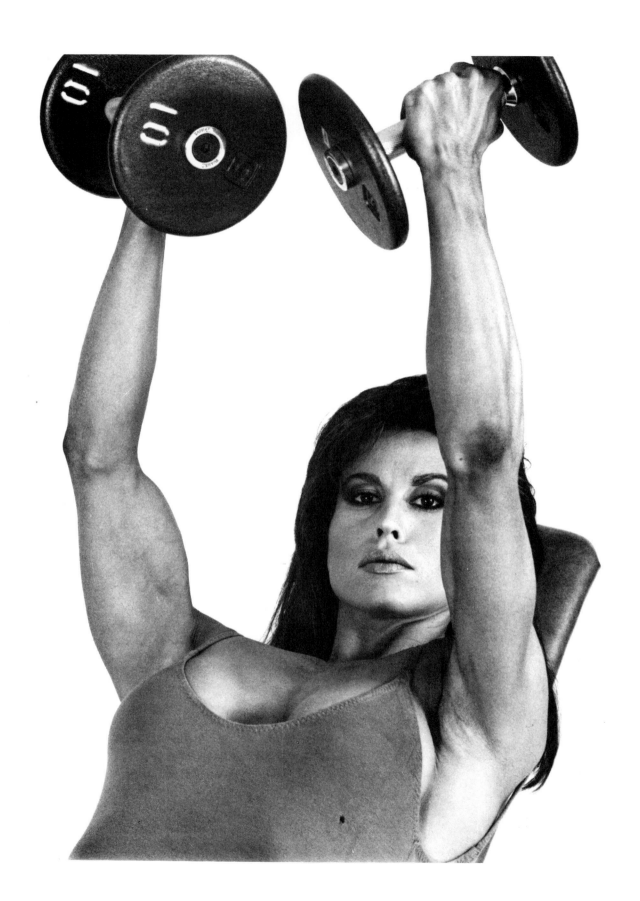

11

The <u>Perfect Parts</u> Triceps Routine

The triceps is probably the most neglected muscle on the human body, especially on women. It doesn't come into play that often in doing the work required for normal, everyday living. To locate your own triceps muscle, extend your arm straight out from your side. Now look at the part of your arm that runs from your elbow to just under your armpit. That's your triceps muscle. Is it loose or tight? If it's very loose, you'll wonder, "Could this be a muscle? It seems more like hanging skin or fat and skin."

Out-of-shape triceps greatly detract from the overall balance and beauty of the feminine physique. A woman can be in perfect physical condition, but if her triceps are soft and flabby, she immediately adds the look of aging to her overall appearance. Loose triceps are one of the first signs commonly associated with getting older. But don't be discouraged. Most women do not have well-developed triceps unless they do specific exercises to develop that muscle. But here's the good news: It's relatively easy to develop the triceps.

Because the triceps is a smaller muscle than most others, it requires less stimulation in order to shape up. Instead of doing five exercises for your triceps, as you did with chest and shoulders, you only need to do three.

Drooping, sagging triceps are the result of a combination of neglect and the natural atrophy of muscle that comes with inactivity—not necessarily with age. You can make quick work of shaping your triceps muscle by following the simple routine presented in this chapter.

You will never have to worry about overdeveloping your triceps. The muscle responds well to weight training, but it responds at a slow, steady pace. In order to have overdeveloped triceps muscles, you would have to do tons of work on them, using methods not covered in this book.

When working on your triceps muscle, you'll quickly discover that it is extremely important to do the exercise strictly and to concentrate fully. While this is true with every exercise you do for all body parts, the triceps requires added concentration because it is so easy to find ways to avoid working the muscle. Since you're probably not used to working that area of your body, your body will attempt to avoid the work by using other muscles to help do the work. For this reason you must be sure to catch yourself every time you start cheating by using momentum or other body parts to help you in the exercise. It doesn't really matter how light you have to go in the beginning in order to do the exercise correctly. The crucial issue is whether you are performing the exercise in perfect form and getting maximum contraction on each movement.

THE TRICEPS MUSCLE

The triceps muscle consists of three parts—that's why the name is in the plural form, "triceps" and not "tricep." One of the three heads of this muscle attaches to the shoulder blade. The other two heads have their origin at the inside of the humerus and are connected near the elbow joint. The triceps works to extend the forearm and the arm in general and to help pull the arm back once it has been extended.

The three heads of the triceps are the inner head, the outer head, and the medial head. Most women are in serious need of inner triceps work, so we have included a tailormade exercise sequence for this area.

DEVELOPMENT

The triceps often take a bit longer than most muscles to develop, but considering the small amount of exercise you have to do in order to develop them, you get a lot for your exercise time. You should see results anywhere between two and five months, but your triceps will feel tighter after your very first workout.

EXERCISES

There are three exercises for your triceps workout. If you are working at home, follow the home list. (These exercises are presented first.) If you are working out in a gym or a fitness center, follow the gym list. (These exercises are presented after the home exercises.)

HOME TRICEPS ROUTINE

1. Seated two-arm dumbbell triceps extension
2. Dumbbell kickback
3. Cross-face triceps extension

GYM TRICEPS ROUTINE

1. Seated two-arm dumbbell triceps extension
2. Pulley push-down
3. Cross-face triceps extension

Do seven to eleven repetitions for each of your three sets. If you find that you cannot get at least seven repetitions for your set, you have selected too heavy a weight. If you find that you are getting eleven repetitions too easily, you have selected too light a weight. Raise your weight once it gets too easy (usually after about a month).

HOW OFTEN TO WORK OUT

Work your triceps every other day or three times a week, unless you are on a four-day split routine, working your entire body. Then you will work your triceps only twice a week.

WARM-UP/PRE-STRETCH

Extend both arms directly up over your head, then bend your left arm at the elbow and touch the palm of your left hand to the back of your neck (or, if you're really flexible, your upper back). With your other hand, gently press the bent elbow against your head, at the same time bending slightly to the right from the waist. Hold the stretch for five seconds. Repeat this three times, then extend both arms again and do the same on the right side.

This brief movement will stretch your triceps in preparation for a light warm-up set to precede the routine that follows.

126

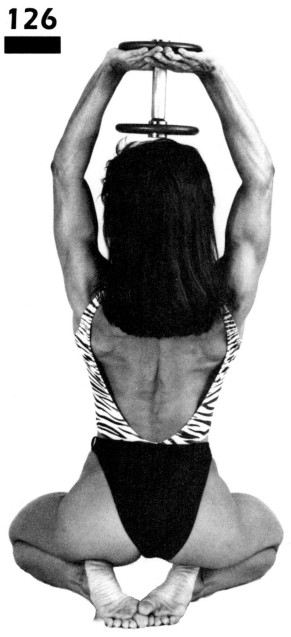

Start

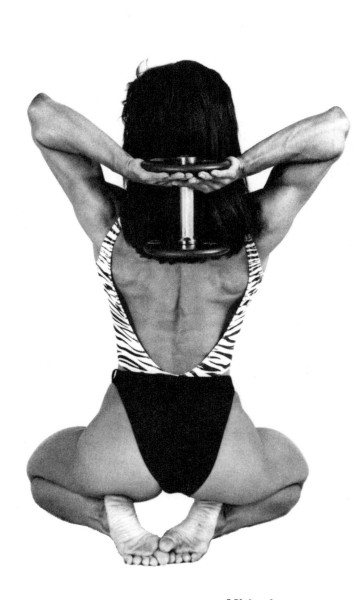

Midpoint

HOME TRICEPS ROUTINE

Seated Two-Arm Triceps Extension

This exercise works to develop the entire triceps area, especially the inner and middle heads of the muscle.

POSITIONING

- Sit on the floor or on a flat exercise bench (legs astride the bench, feet on the floor) holding a dumbbell in both hands between your crossed thumbs and fingers. Your palms should be facing you.
- Extend your arms straight up, keeping your biceps as close to the side of your head as possible. Look straight ahead.

THE MOVEMENT

- Lower the dumbbell behind your head until it touches your upper back. Feel the stretch in your triceps area.
- Flex your triceps as you return to start position.
- Repeat the movement until you have completed your set.

REMEMBER

- Don't push the dumbbell up in an uncontrolled fashion. Concentrate and maintain a fluid movement.
- Maintain control of the dumbbell on the downward movement.

VARIATION

- You can do this exercise one arm at a time. (Use the free hand to ensure control in good, strict form.)
- Alternate arms, doing a full number of sets for either side.

128   **Start**

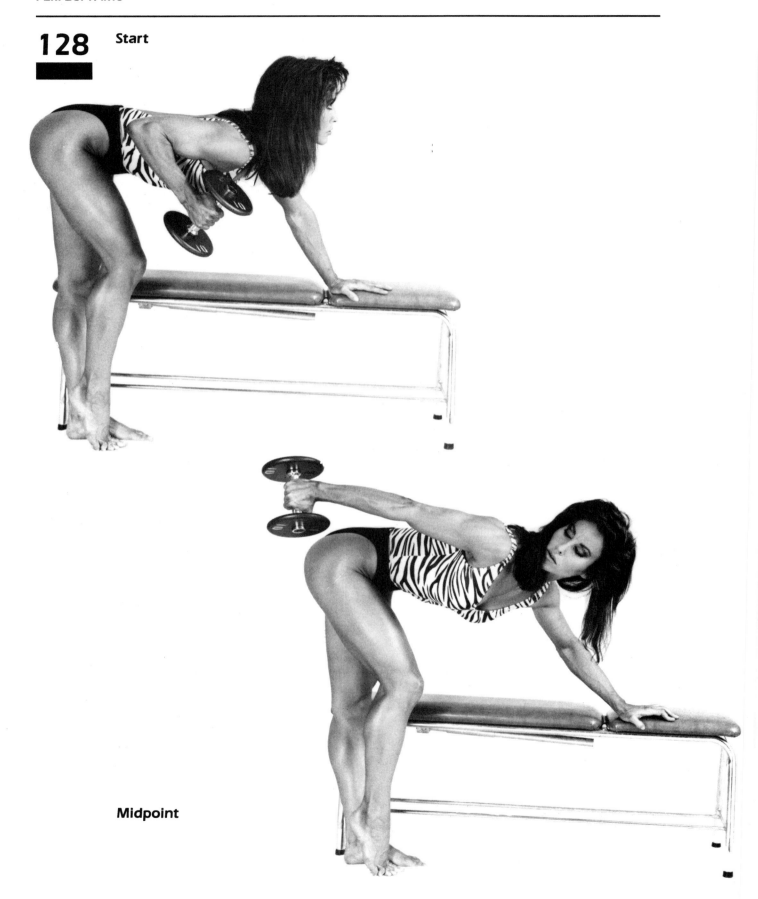

Midpoint

Dumbbell Kickback

Dumbbell kickbacks perfect the entire triceps area, especially the outer head of the muscle.

POSITIONING

■ Grasp a dumbbell in your right hand, palm facing your body, and lean over until your torso is parallel to the floor. (Stand with the side of your body to the mirror so that you can see your triceps muscle.)
■ Holding your elbow against your waist, bend your arm so that your forearm is parallel to the floor.

THE MOVEMENT

■ Extend your arm down and back in a semicircle until it is fully extended behind you, or "kicked back," flexing your triceps muscle throughout the movement.
■ Experience the peak contraction for a moment in the fully extended position.
■ Return to start position and feel the stretch as you bend your arm fully.
■ Repeat the movement until you have completed your set.
■ Repeat the set for your left arm.

REMEMBER

■ Keep your elbow against your waist at all times.
■ Control the dumbbell throughout the movement. Be careful not to swing it.

130

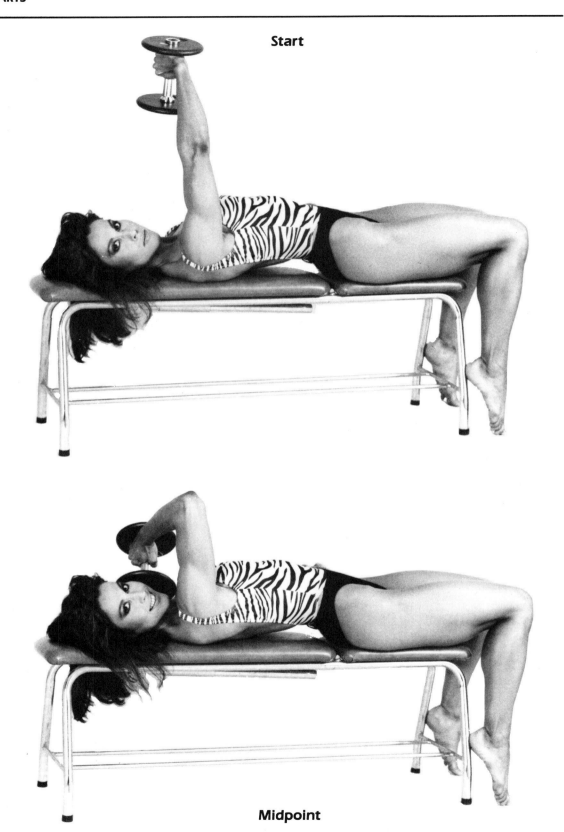

Start

Midpoint

Cross-Face Triceps Extension

This exercise perfects the inner triceps area, which is the most neglected part of the triceps muscle.

POSITIONING

■ Grasp a dumbbell in your right arm and lie on a flat exercise bench or on the floor.

■ Extend your right arm straight up, holding the dumbbell with your palm directly forward. Turn your face toward your arm so that your chin is just about touching your shoulder.

THE MOVEMENT

■ Bending your arm at the elbow, lower the dumbbell until the edge of it grazes your *left* ear. Feel the stretch in your triceps area.

■ Flex your triceps as you return to the start position.

■ Repeat the movement until you have completed your set.

■ Perform the next set with your other arm, and continue to alternate right and left arms until you have completed three sets for either side.

REMEMBER

■ Your arm will be moving downward, across your face for each repetition. Be sure to keep your face averted to the side throughout the exercise. (You can also reduce risk of injury by using your free hand to "spot" for the working arm throughout the movement. But be sure you don't cheat while doing so.)

■ Concentrate on flexing your triceps on the up movement and stretching them on the down movement.

132 GYM TRICEPS ROUTINE

Seated Two-Arm Dumbbell Triceps Extension

Follow the instructions on page 127.

Pulley Push-down

Pulley push-downs perfect the entire triceps muscle, especially the outer area.

POSITIONING

■ Place your hands, palms down, four to eight inches apart on the pulley push-down bar.
■ Bend at the elbows and fully extend your forearms upward.
■ Pin your upper arms to your body throughout the exercise.

THE MOVEMENT

■ Push the bar down until your arms are completely extended downward. Flex (squeeze) your triceps and return to the start position, remaining in full control of the weights.
■ Repeat the movement until you have completed your set.

REMEMBER

■ Be careful to keep your elbows at your sides throughout the movement. Don't let them lift on the upward movement
■ Do the work with your triceps muscles, not with your shoulders or back.
■ Resist the temptation to lean forward and push the bar away from your body in an effort to make the work easier. Maintain perfect form throughout the exercise, since it takes perfect form to develop perfect parts.
■ Stretch your triceps again after completing the exercise.

Cross-Face Triceps Extension

Follow the instructions on page 131.

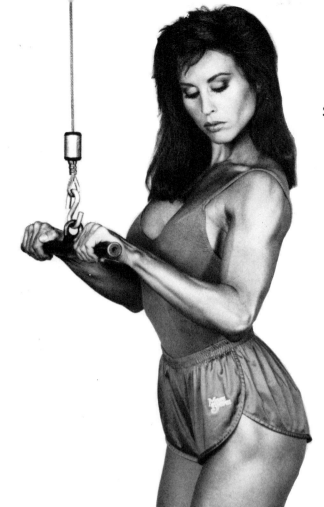

Start

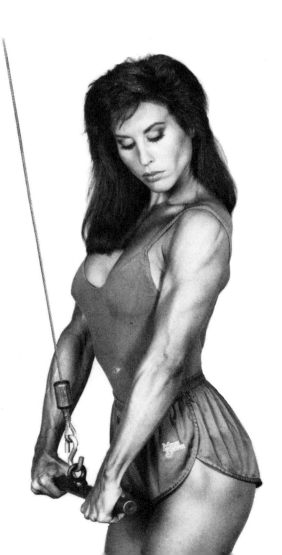

Midpoint

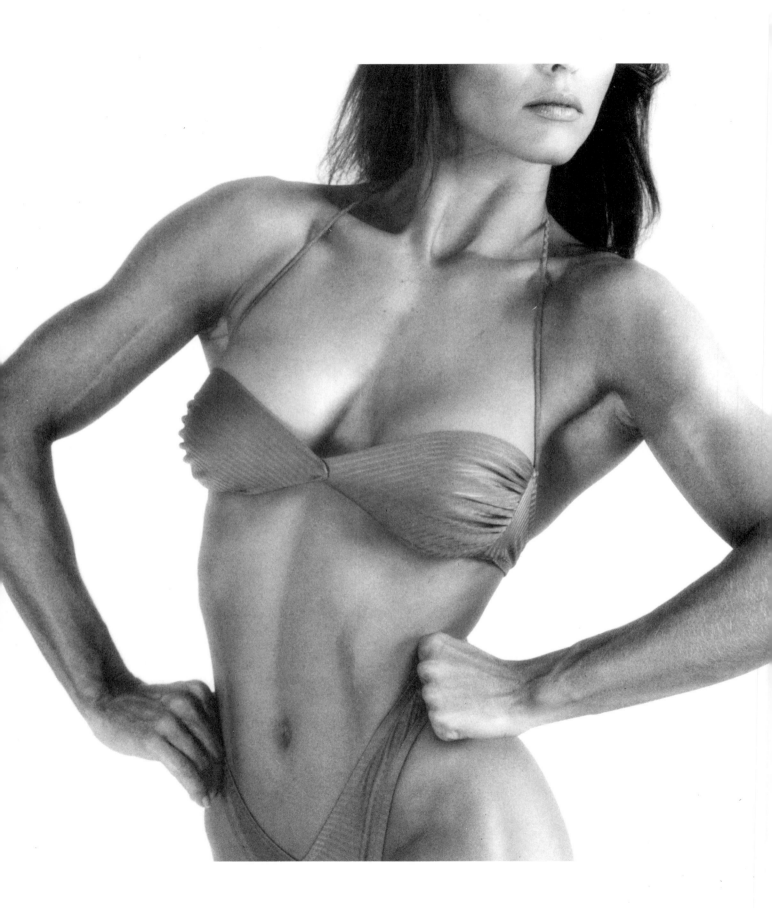

12

The _Perfect Parts_ Abdominal Routine

No one would argue that the abdominal or stomach area takes the prize for being a problem to most people, and for this reason it is usually the best place to start if you are considering working only one or two body parts. A flat, tight abdominal area will give you a much more positive feeling about your entire body.

The stomach or abdominal area is a favorite place for fat to accumulate, and if you are even a few pounds overweight and your abdominal muscles are weak, your stomach will protrude. You'll want to diet (see chapter 16) if you are overweight and want to see results. Otherwise, even though you'll develop fine muscles on your stomach after carefully following this routine, you'll never see them. The fat that remains will obscure them. The fat is still what you'll see, although it probably won't protrude quite as much as before.

If you follow this routine, not only will you have a flat, toned stomach with sculpted contours of definition, but you'll also build yourself a natural girdle of muscle so that you have no trouble at all holding your stomach in.

There's hardly a woman alive who would argue the need to work on her stomach. Even ladies with flat stomachs like to do some exercise in that area, just to make sure their stomach stays flat.

136

THE ABDOMINAL MUSCLES

The rectus abdominis is the primary abdominal muscle. Contrary to popular belief, it doesn't have separate upper and lower parts. It is a long, slender muscle that runs vertically up and down across your abdominal wall. It has a right and left half, separated by a tendonous strip called the linea alba.

The misconception regarding "upper" and "lower" aspects of the rectus abdominis arises from the fact that some abdominal exercises do not contract the entire muscle fully. Depending on the exercise, you feel the contraction more in the upper or lower portion of the muscle.

Another abdominal area, one usually not given much attention, is comprised of the "obliques," both external and internal. The external and internal obliques run at an angle along the sides and front of the abdomen. The obliques slant toward each other and form the hollow of the waist where they intersect. The greater the natural slant, the smaller the waist of the individual, assuming absence of flabby fat there. The only real way to work the oblique muscles is to do twisting motions as in the serratus crunch exercise described for this workout.

DEVELOPMENT

Assuming you are not more than 5 pounds overweight, you should begin to see some abdominal development after about two months of working out. In four months you'll see definition beginning to form, and in six months you'll begin to feel that natural girdle of sculpted muscle building up underneath your stomach. You'll be able to hold your stomach in without much effort. In a year you'll have a perfectly formed, sensual abdominal area.

ABDOMINAL AWARENESS

If your abdominal area has been totally neglected over the years, and you have not developed a basic abdominal awareness, I'd like to let you in on a little secret to help you begin to hold your stomach in, even if you are now significantly overweight. Wear a belt *under* your clothing. It should be a thin and comfortable belt—the stretchy exercise belts are best—but make it tight enough so that you know it is there. The belt should fit unnoticeably under your clothing, on your bare skin. Wearing the belt will remind you to begin to use your own natural muscles to hold your abdominal area in rather than let it all hang out. If you decide to wear a belt this way and learn to use it as a reminder to pull your stomach in, then once you have exercised your abdominal area for a few months you will be that much ahead of the game. You will have acquired "ab awareness." You will have acquired the habit of flexing or controlling your stomach muscles, and the simple act of flexing or holding in the stomach itself helps to tighten muscles.

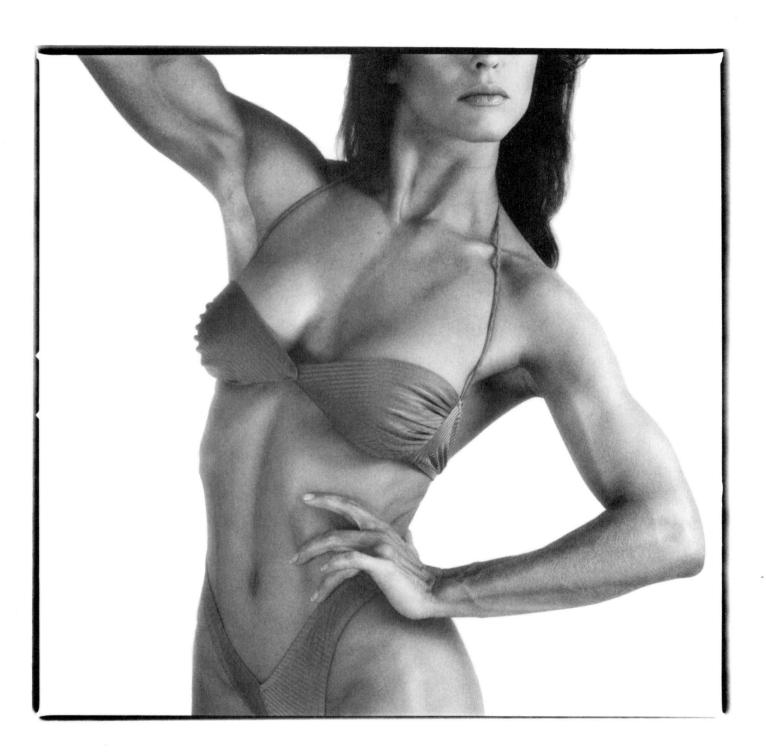

EXERCISES

There are five exercises for the abdominal area. You will follow the same routine, whether you are working at home or in a gym or fitness center.

HOME AND GYM ABDOMINAL ROUTINE

1. Standard sit-up
2. Crunch
3. Serratus crunch
4. Knee-up leg-up combination
5. Bent-knee leg lift

REPETITIONS

The abdominals require the most repetitions of movement for development. Try to build up to the point where you can do three sets of twenty-five repetitions for each set of each exercise. Since you may not have worked your abdominals in a long time (maybe you never worked them) you can break in slowly. The first day, just do as many reps for each set as you can, and then take it from there.

Once in a while, just to test yourself, go wild and do as many reps as you can for the last set of an abdominal exercise. This will build strength, muscle endurance, and confidence, and it breaks up the routine.

ADDING ANKLE WEIGHTS TO YOUR ROUTINE

After you have achieved the goal of three sets of twenty-five repetitions for each of your abdominal exercises, you can add ankle weights to your routine. You will note that the only exercises for which ankle weights or dumbbells would be practical are knee-ups and leg-ups. Sit-ups and crunches would not be affected by adding weights, as you will see once you begin your workout.

Purchase ankle bracelets that allow you to add weights through slotted openings, so that you can begin with 1 pound and work your way up as high as 3 pounds per leg. You can also use a light dumbbell (3 or 5 pounds) instead of ankle weights.

HOW OFTEN TO WORK OUT

Work your abdominal area at least two times a week. You can also choose to perform this routine every other day. There's really no need to work your abdominals every day, but if you really want to, be sure to give yourself at least one day off a week.

I think it's wasted energy to work your abdominal area more than every other day—it's just not efficient. You could be spending that extra time working other neglected body parts. Better yet, take a brisk two- to four-mile walk, run, or bike ride. This will do more for your waistline—by helping to burn off the fat around it—than another several sets of abdominal exercises. While it takes exercise to sculpt those perfect muscles you desire, it takes aerobic exercise and diet to trim away excess weight. Sure, you'll burn off some calories while doing your abdominal exercises, but for the real difference—one you can see within a matter of weeks—be sure also to perform an aerobic activity regularly and cut back on calorie intake.

WARM-UP/PRE-STRETCH

You will need a bar or stick (a broom handle works perfectly) for this seated twisting movement, which may be familiar to you already. Not only is this a great warm-up/pre-stretch movement, but it actually works to tighten the sides of your waist.

Sit on the edge of a stool or flat exercise bench and plant your feet firmly on the floor at more than shoulder width (to keep your lower body stationary throughout the movement). Place the bar or stick across the top of your back and wrap your arms around it in a forward direction. Holding your arms in that position, twist your torso rhythmically and forcibly as far to the left and then the right as you can. Do this for about two minutes.

140 ABDOMINAL ROUTINE

Standard Sit-up

Sit-ups perfect the upper abdominal area.

POSITIONING

- Lie flat on your back on the floor or an exercise mat.
- Bend your knees to approximately a 30-degree angle (to ensure proper support for your spine throughout the movement) and cross your arms in front of your chest.

THE MOVEMENT

- Begin the sit-up by raising your head up off the floor or exercise mat.
- Then lift your shoulders, upper back, and lower back from the floor or mat in progression in a curl-up manner.
- Maintaining continuous tension, uncurl your body all the way to the start position.
- Repeat the movement without resting until you have completed your set.

REMEMBER

- You may be tempted to spring off the floor in an effort to avoid stressing your abdominal muscles. The goal is to achieve peak contraction, to force your abdominal muscles to work, not to find ways to save them from working.
- Do not rest when you return to start. Forget the fact that you are lying on the floor—this is not the time to relax. Keep going until you finish your set.

Start

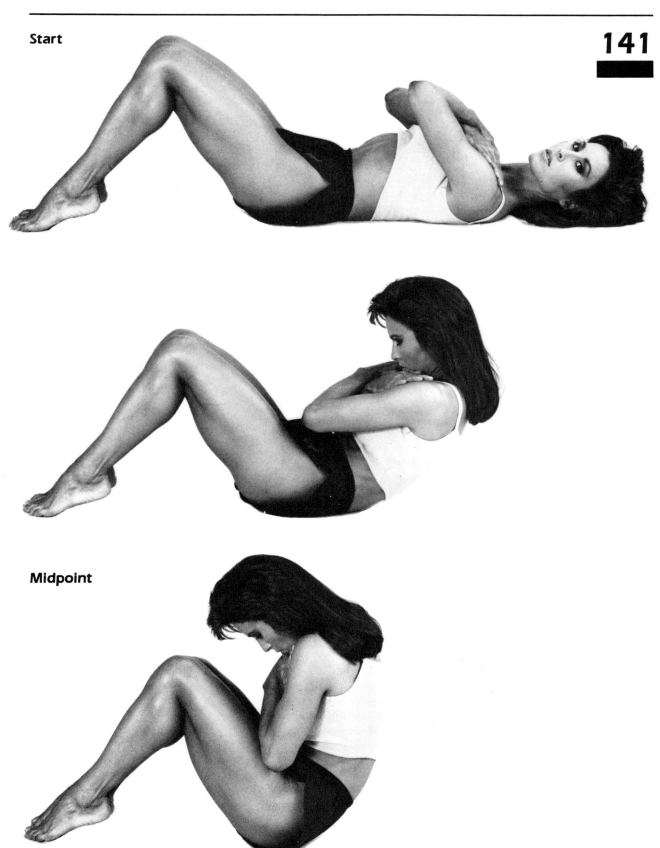

Midpoint

142 Start

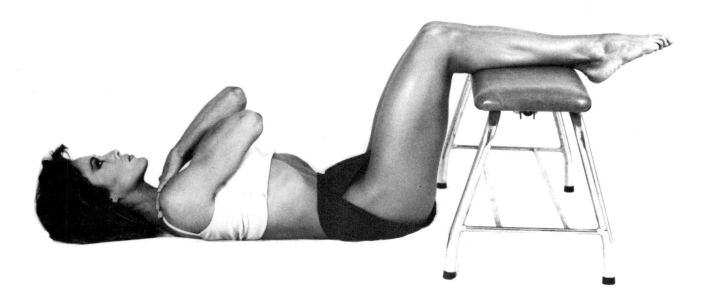

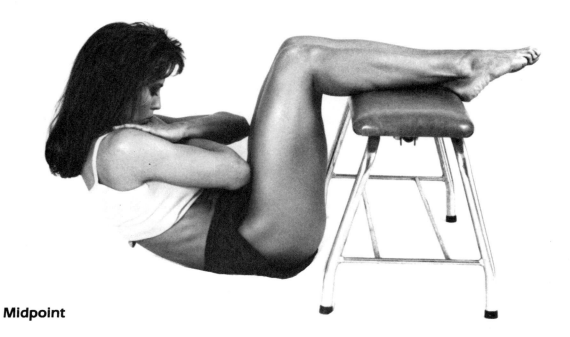

Midpoint

Crunch

This exercise also perfects the upper abdominal area.

POSITIONING

- Lie flat on your back on the floor or an exercise mat and place your legs over a flat exercise bench so that your thighs are perpendicular to the floor.
- Cross your hands on your chest.

THE MOVEMENT

- Take a deep breath and then exhale as you slowly curl your body up, lifting your head first, then your shoulders and upper torso. Keep your mind focused on your upper abdominals throughout the exercise.
- Raise yourself high enough to lift your upper body one-third of the way to your knees.
- Lower yourself to start position without losing tension on your abdominal area.
- Repeat the movement without resting until you have completed your set.

REMEMBER

- Resist the temptation to spring off the floor and throw your head forward in an effort to take pressure off the working abdominal muscles.
- Do not raise your body higher than shoulder height or you will lose some of the effect on your abdominal muscles.
- Don't rest when you return to start.
- An exaggerated inhalation/exhalation breathing pattern will help you achieve a superior contraction.

144 Start

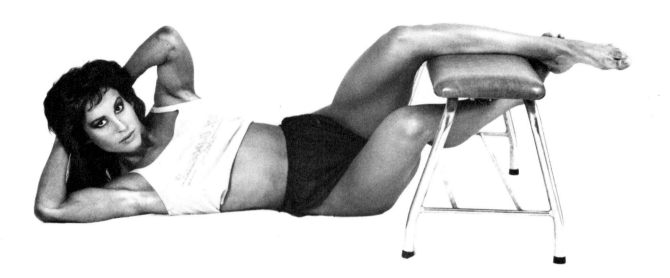

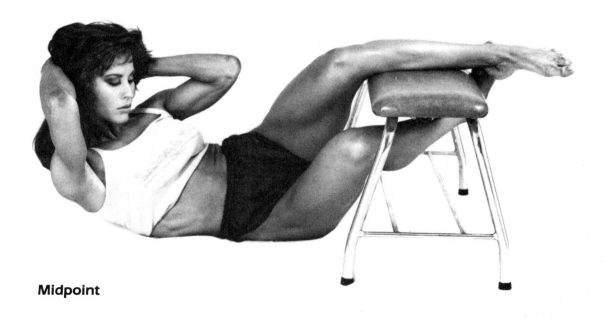

Midpoint

Serratus Crunch

145

The serratus crunch perfects both the upper abdominal area and the intercostals.

POSITIONING

- Lie flat on your back on the floor or an exercise mat.
- Wrap your legs around a flat exercise bench, placing your right leg over the bench and your left leg under the bench and crossing your legs at the ankles.
- Clasp your hands behind your neck.

THE MOVEMENT

- Raise yourself up on your right side by lifting your shoulders and torso until you feel an intense contraction in your waist. Return to start position and repeat the movement without resting until you have completed your set.
- Reverse the position of your legs and repeat the exercise for your left side.
- Repeat the exercise until you have done three sets for either side of your body.

REMEMBER

- Keep your mind riveted on your frontal abs and oblique (side) abdominal muscles.
- Forcefully exhale as you lift up.
- Resist the temptation to lurch wildly off the floor in an effort to gain momentum and make the work easier. Work steadily and with total concentration.
- Keep your abdominal muscles flexed throughout the movement.

146 Start   Midpoint

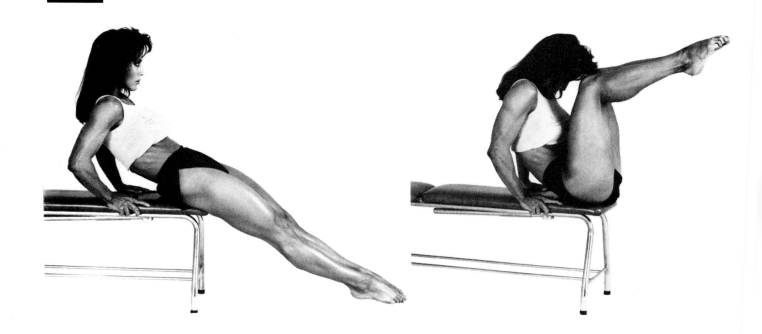

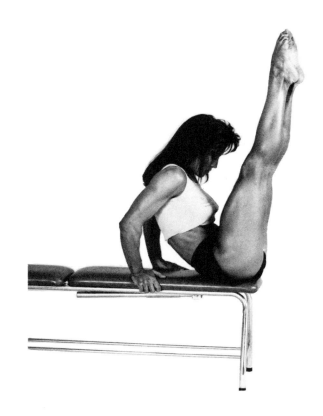

Variation

Knee-up Leg-up Combination

147

This combination exercise perfects the entire abdominal wall but particularly the lower abdominal area. It also stimulates the muscles that flex the hip area.

POSITIONING

- Lie on the floor on your back and place your hands under your hips.
- Lift your head and tuck your chin into your chest.
- Raise the heels of your feet two inches off the floor.

THE MOVEMENT

- Concentrating on your lower abdominal muscles, bend your legs fully and aim your knees at your forehead. (Don't be discouraged if your knees do not reach your forehead. Just raise them as close to your face as possible. In time you will be able to get them up close.)
- Remain in this position for a few seconds while flexing your abdominal muscles, then slowly return to start.
- Without letting your heels touch the ground, repeat the movement until you have completed your set.

REMEMBER

- Don't let your mind wander away from your abdominal muscles. Continually flex (squeeze) them and make them do the work.
- Control your movement both ways, up and down. Never let your legs simply drop to the start position. Never forget: Perfect movements for perfect parts.

VARIATION

- Extend your legs straight up from the bent-knee position and slowly lower them to the start position.
- Flex your buttocks as you lower your legs.

148

Start

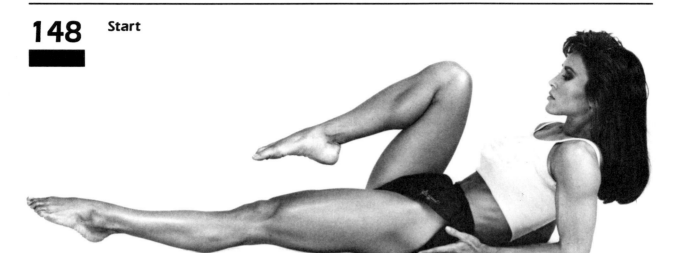

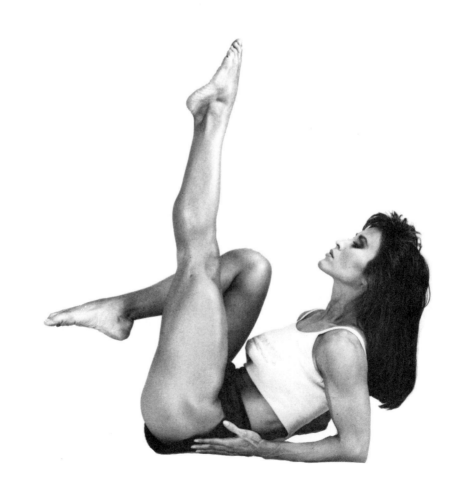

Midpoint

Bent-Knee Leg Lift

This exercise perfects the entire abdominal area and also stimulates the sartorius and rectus femoris muscles in the legs.

POSITIONING

■ Lie on the floor or an exercise mat and raise yourself up by supporting your body with your elbows.

■ Bend your right leg as much as you can and hold it just over your abdominal area. Let it remain in that position throughout the exercise. This prevents strain on the lower back during the movement. (If you find it difficult to achieve this position, let your foot rest on the floor, keeping the leg as bent as possible.)

■ Extend your left leg straight out in front of you, toes pointed straight ahead, and raise the heel of your foot two inches off the floor. Keep your left leg straight as you perform the exercise.

THE MOVEMENT

■ Raise your left leg until it is perpendicular to the floor. Be careful not to move your other leg at all.

■ Return to start position, being sure not to let your heel touch the floor.

■ Repeat the movement without resting until you have completed your set. Work up to twenty-five reps.

■ Repeat the set for your other leg.

REMEMBER

■ Try not to rock back and forth during the exercise. (It takes a little time to learn the balance of this exercise. Don't worry, you'll get it right before you know it.)

■ Keep concentrating on your abdominal muscles. Think "tight tummy!"

■ Flex your lower abdominal muscles throughout the movement, especially as you forcefully exhale while raising your leg.

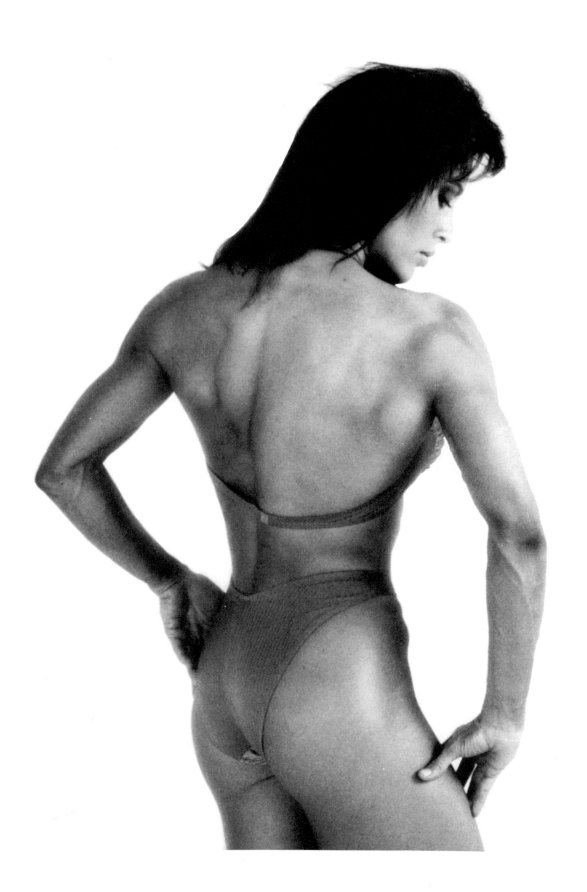

13

The __Perfect Parts__ Buttocks-Hip Routine

Why are we women so critical of our behinds? I've noticed that even women who have buttocks that others admire insist that they can't stand their butts and wish to reshape them.

Whether your buttocks are in really bad shape or whether you don't like your buttocks even though you know you can get by with them the way they are, we have developed a routine for you that will once and for all reshape, firm, tone, solidify, and lift that dreaded part of your anatomy. You'll see it for yourself—clearly.

In order to assist you in seeing, we suggest that you have someone take "rear view" pictures of you in a bathing suit and in pants; then hide the pictures somewhere for three months. Then take another picture. Wow! You'll be very surprised to see the change. You can take such a picture every three months for a year, and if you follow this routine strictly, we guarantee you'll continue to see positive changes in your buttocks.

We don't have to tell you that out-of-shape buttocks throw the body out of balance. Even viewed from the front, your hips appear wider when your buttocks are out of proportion. Viewed from the rear, large or sagging buttocks make a woman look dumpy and even comical.

Some women avoid dealing with the issue by refusing to look in the mirror at their buttocks. One of us did this for years—you can guess who—and was horrified when finally she looked around to see the reality. Fortunately she did something about it.

Genetics do play a part in the shape of your buttocks. Some women have naturally bigger gluteus maximus areas than others. These women will always have a large

151

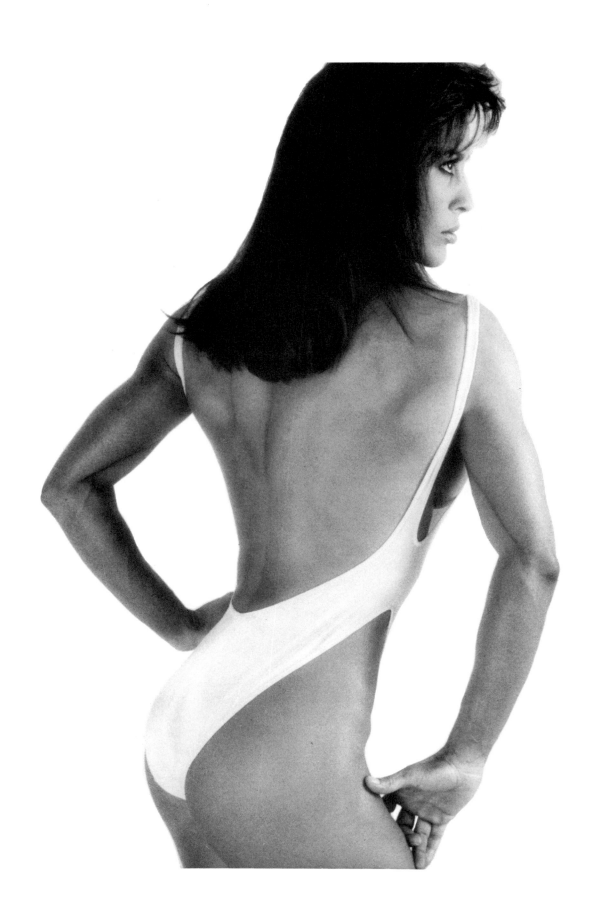

buttocks area, but they can tighten, shape, and tone the buttocks to be more appealing, even attractive. But it does require doing the work.

THE BUTTOCKS AND HIP MUSCLES

The buttock muscle, the gluteus maximus, is located behind the hip joint. It is the largest muscle on your body—and a very obvious muscle by virtue of its protruding position. It works to rotate the thigh, to give momentum for strenuous movements such as climbing, squatting, or darting, and to extend the upper thigh from the hip joint.

The hip muscles consist of the other two, smaller gluteus muscles, the gluteus medius and the gluteus minimus. The gluteus medius rises from the hipbone just under the gluteus maximus. It works to raise the leg outward and sideways and to give balance when transferring weight from one leg to the other. The gluteus medius originates toward the front part of the hipbone and inserts in front of the gluteus medius on the thighbone. It also raises the leg outward and sideways and helps to balance the body when shifting weight.

All exercises in the routine given here work primarily to shape the gluteus maximus, but the gluteus medius and the gluteus minimus are affected positively, too.

DEVELOPMENT

It takes a while to see results in the hip-buttocks area. To begin with, a woman's center of gravity is lower than a man's, and her pelvis is proportionately wider. This is connected with the biology of pregnancy and childbirth. So to try to narrow the hip-buttocks area is to wrestle with nature itself. But we can still minimize our maximus spread if we work at it. And then there is the fact that fat likes to accumulate on this area, perhaps because our buttocks serve us as a natural cushion when sitting down. It seems as if the Creator was more concerned with safety, function, and comfort than with our vanity.

While you can count on seeing some results in three months, don't expect reshaped buttocks until at least six months. It may take as long as a year to achieve really perfect buttocks.

If you are overweight, chances are it will take a little longer to see your completely reshaped buttocks, because fat likes to accumulate there. But as the fat slowly melts away, you will be able to see your newly reshaped, uplifted, muscular buttocks. Be patient and remember to visualize and cooperate with yourself by using your mind as an ally.

EXERCISES

There are five exercises for the hips-buttocks area. You will do the same routine whether you are working at home or in a gym or fitness center.

HOME AND GYM BUTTOCKS-HIP ROUTINE

1. Standing hip hyperextension
2. Pelvic lift
3. Single-leg buttocks tightener
4. Lunge
5. Double-leg buttocks tightener

REPETITIONS

Your buttocks comprise a very large muscle group. Twenty repetitions for each set of each exercise is the ideal amount for best results. If you are not used to exercising this area, don't push yourself too hard in the beginning. Just do as many reps as you can for each set until you work your way up to the suggested number of reps for each exercise. This may take you a couple of weeks or months. Set weekly goals. Say to yourself, "I got seven reps per set this week; next week I'll get ten reps per set," and then make yourself do it. Easy does it and before you know it you'll be doing the full program. Then it will be time for another challenge.

ADDING ANKLE WEIGHTS TO YOUR ROUTINE

After you have achieved the goal of three sets of twenty repetitions for each exercise, you can add ankle weights. You may already have purchased them for your abdominal routine. If not, buy ankle bracelets that have slots for adding weight. You should begin with 1-pound weights for each leg and build up to about 3 pounds. No need to go much higher than that.

HOW OFTEN TO WORK OUT

You should work your buttocks at least two times a week or you can choose to work them every other day. There's no need to work any more than that.

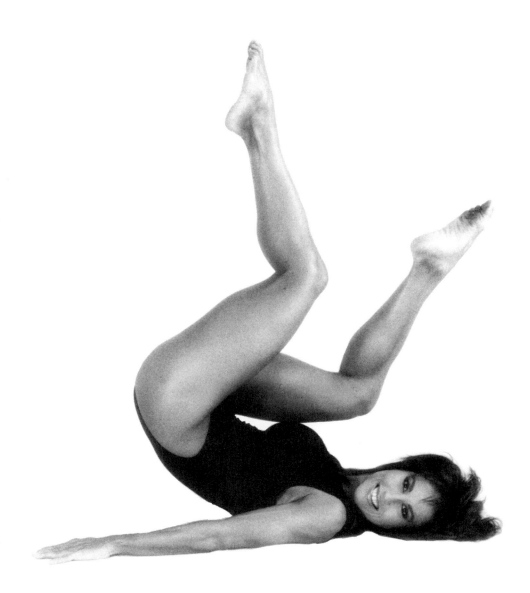

WARM-UP/PRE-STRETCH

Lie on the floor, flat on your back, and raise your hips up in the air, holding them up by keeping your shoulder-to-elbow area flat on the floor and supporting your waist–hip area with your hands. Now ride the bicycle: Wheel your legs around in a circular motion, ten times in one direction and ten in the other. You may want to do this for two or three minutes if you're having fun. Try to bring your legs as close to your chest as possible each time you wheel around.

Now, if—and only if—you are flexible . . . keeping this position, extend your legs straight up in the air, then slowly bring them down *behind* you until you touch the floor behind your head. This will stretch your spine and your buttocks.

If you're not all that flexible, sit on the floor with your legs straight out in front of you. Then bend forward, grasp your ankles, and hold that position to the count of ten. Repeat three times.

156

Start

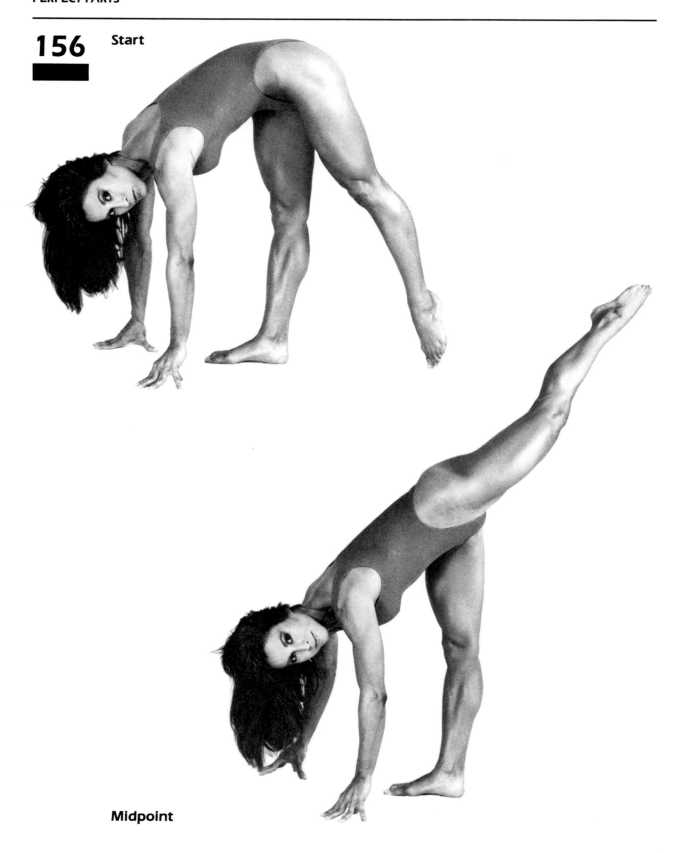

Midpoint

BUTTOCKS-HIPS ROUTINE

Standing Hip Hyperextension

This exercise tightens and uplifts the gluteus maximus (buttocks) muscles, tightens and narrows the hips, and strengthens the lower back.

POSITIONING

- Stand with your feet a natural width apart and lean forward, bending over until your fingertips touch the floor roughly a foot or two in front of your feet.
- Extend your left leg straight back, keeping your toes pointed as well.

THE MOVEMENT

- Keeping your torso angled straight to the floor at about 45 degrees, lift your left leg behind you, forming a tripod with your right leg and two arms.
- Keeping your left leg as stiff as a board, lift it behind you as high as possible and simultaneously flex (squeeze) your left buttocks-hip area as hard as possible.
- Slowly return to start and, without resting, repeat the movement until you have completed your set.
- Perform the movement for the right leg.
- Repeat the exercise until you have completed three sets for each leg.

REMEMBER

- Do not allow the knee of the working leg to bend; keep it flexed and tight.
- Keep the nonworking leg as straight as possible, but don't "lock out" your knee.
- Flex your buttocks-hip area throughout the exercise, especially at the top of the movement.
- Do not become discouraged if you lose your balance or feel awkward in the beginning, or if you can't lift your leg very high. In time you will become adjusted to this movement.
- Maintain perfect form to ensure proper peak contraction.

VARIATION

- You can do this exercise from an "all fours" position.
- While kneeling on a mat or padded surface, place your weight on your right knee, then bend your left knee and bring it to your chest.
- Follow by extending your left leg behind you as high as possible while flexing your hip-buttocks area with all your strength.
- Return to start position and repeat the movement until you have finished your set.
- Repeat the exercise for your right buttocks-hip area.

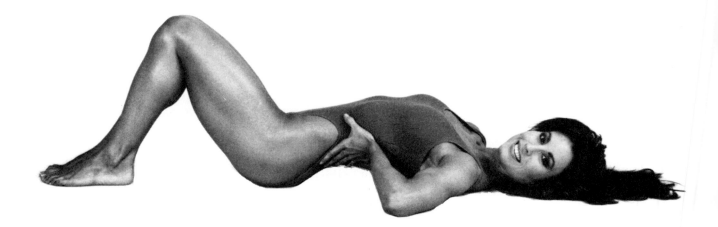

Start

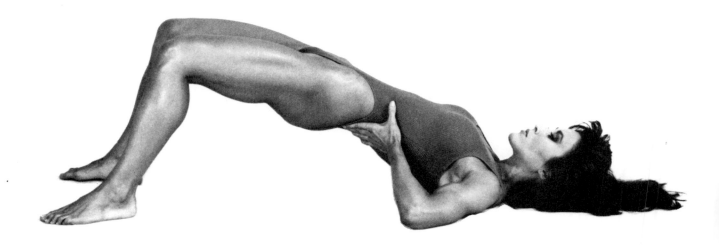

Midpoint

Pelvic Lift

Pelvic lifts perfect the entire buttocks area and the lower back, strengthening the erector spinae muscles in particular.

POSITIONING

- Lie flat on your back on a padded floor or mat.
- Raise your knees and position your feet on the floor somewhat back toward your buttocks.
- Support yourself by placing your hands at the small of your back so you can feel your erector spinae muscles work and get firm with every rep.

THE MOVEMENT

- Raise your buttocks off the floor as high as possible while flexing (squeezing) your glutes with all your strength.
- When you've raised yourself to the highest possible point, give your buttocks an extra hard squeeze.
- Return to start and relax for a split second.
- Repeat the up/down movement until you have completed your set. (Work up to a set of twenty-five reps.)
- For muscle contraction specificity you can vary the positioning of your feet.

REMEMBER

- Keep your feet on the floor throughout the movement.
- Control the squeeze, and really feel the flex in your glutes.

VARIATION

- Hold the up position on the fifteenth rep, and bring your feet and knees together for an additional five reps.
- Then, keeping your feet together but separating your knees wide, do ten more reps.
- Bring your knees and feet together as before, keeping your bottom as high and flexed as you can at the same time.
- With your hips still raised, scoot your feet to within just a few inches of your body, and slowly bring your hips down to rest for a split second before raising them up again for five last peak contractions. (This will give you an experience of muscle contraction specificity, which you can intensify by extending one leg straight up and supporting it with the other throughout the movement.)

160 Single-Leg Buttocks Tightener

This exercise perfects the entire buttocks area and the erector spinae of the lower back.

POSITIONING

- Lie on the floor, face down, with your arms in a comfortable position crossed or extended in front of you.

THE MOVEMENT

- Flexing your right buttock as hard as possible, lift your right leg behind you as far as possible. (Use your hip area to originate the movement.) Keep your right knee locked throughout the movement.
- Give your right gluteus maximus muscle an extra hard squeeze on the highest point of the movement.
- Return to start and, without resting, repeat the movement until you have completed your set.
- Repeat the exercise for the left buttock.
- You can apply the principle of muscle contraction specificity here, too.

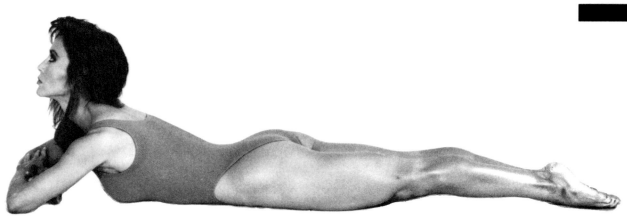

Start

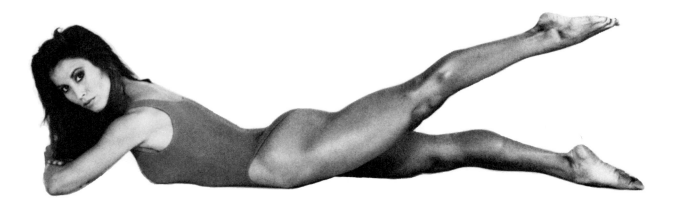

Midpoint

162 **Start**

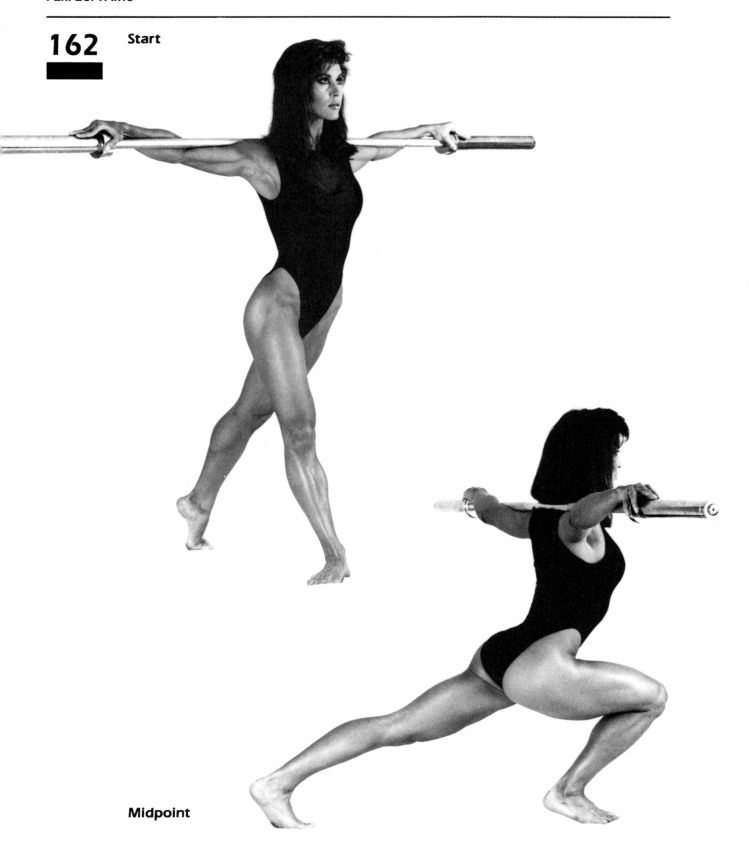

Midpoint

Lunge with Buttocks Squeeze

This movement is great for perfecting the thighs, buttocks, and hip area.

POSITIONING

■ Place a barbell across your shoulders and let it rest on your trapezius muscle, holding it in a wide, comfortable grip.
■ Stand with your feet shoulder width apart and your toes pointed straight ahead.

THE MOVEMENT

■ Keeping your left leg straight, step forward about two to three feet with your right foot.
■ Bend your right knee and, without moving your feet, "lunge" forward as far as you can.
■ At this position, "stretch" the extension of your left leg by tightening and flexing your left buttock and thigh muscles, pushing your left heel toward the floor at the same time.
■ Rise up on your right leg slightly and then lower again for a maximum muscle contraction in the buttock.
■ Raise your left heel to your first point of extension, then return to the start position.
■ Complete your set, then do the movement with the right leg extended back.
■ Alternate legs until you have completed the full number of sets on each side for the exercise.
■ You can apply the muscle contraction specificity principle here to vary the stress.

REMEMBER

■ Since this is a compound movement with a shift in body balance, it's important that you maintain concentration throughout the exercise.

164   Start

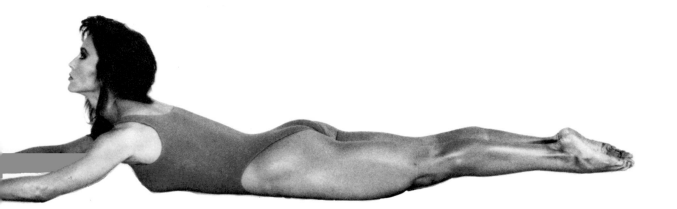

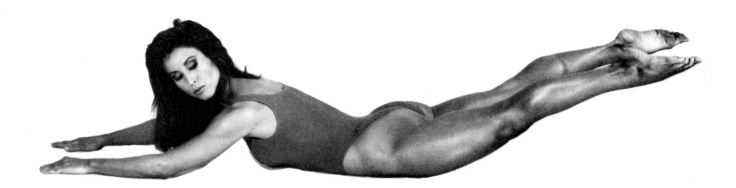

Midpoint

Double-Leg Buttocks Tightener

This exercise variation tightens the entire buttocks area and strengthens the lower back (erector spinae).

POSITIONING AND MOVEMENT

■ Do this movement exactly as the single-leg buttocks tightener, only instead of lifting one leg at a time, lift both legs together, simultaneously flexing the entire buttocks.

■ On the up movement, extend your legs six inches apart in a scissorslike movement and squeeze as hard as you can, then immediately return to start.

■ Repeat the movement until you have finished your set.

VARIATION

■ You can also apply the muscle contraction specificity principle to this movement, as with the single-leg buttocks tightener.

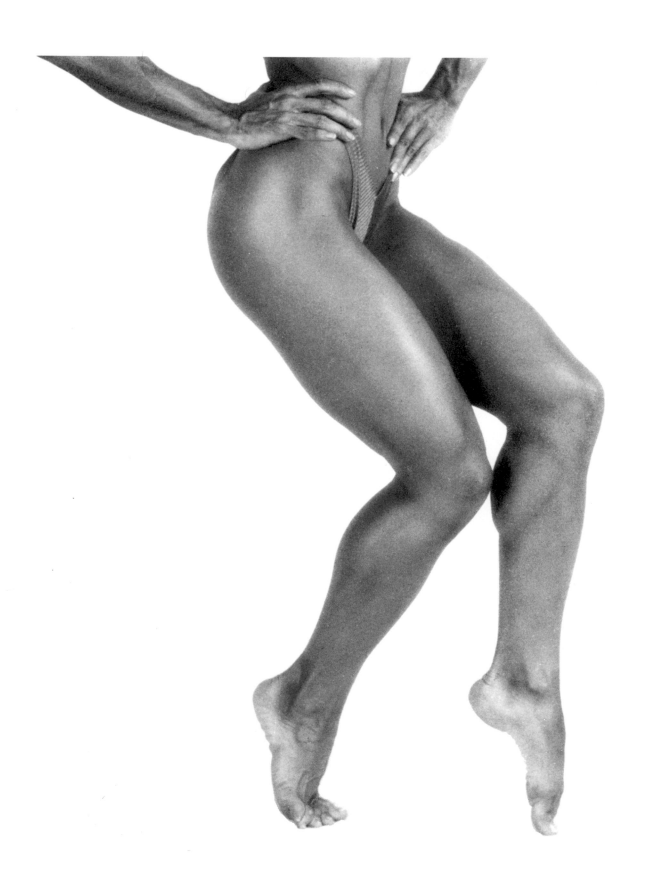

14

The Perfect Parts Thigh Routine

There's absolutely no doubt in my mind. Every woman wants to walk around on a great-looking pair of legs. That means legs that are lean and shapely—gorgeous! Am I right?

Fortunately, great legs are relatively simple to develop. The only secret is that you've got to do some work. But if you're willing to put out the necessary effort, you can possess the kind of legs you think are the exclusive preserve of ballet dancers and gymnasts—or at least come close. Focus on working the muscle groups that produce the most noticeable improvements, and soon you're on your way to the legs of your dreams. In less than a year from now you'll find yourself looking for opportunities to show them off. You may even audition for a stocking commercial!

No matter what condition your thighs are in, work on them. If they are thin, you should place firm muscle under your skin so that your skin will not sag and you will not eventually develop cellulite (fat bunched up on fat because the area is not stimulated by exercise). If you are fat, you should build firm sexy muscle under the fat so that as it melts away you will see a perfectly formed leg emerge. If you already have great legs, this is the way to keep them.

168

THE THIGH MUSCLES

The front thigh consists largely of the quadriceps, four muscles that travel along the front thigh and end in the kneecap: the rectus femoris and three muscles called the "vasti." The basic work of the quadriceps or frontal thigh muscles is to extend the leg from a bent position.

There are three muscles that constitute the back thigh. Together they work to rotate the leg and extend the hips, and they also work to flex the knee. They are located toward the back outside of the thigh and insert through the inside of the knee.

DEVELOPMENT

The thighs, front and back, defy exercise in the beginning stages, or at least they seem to. You will work on your legs for weeks before you see much in the way of results, then suddenly you'll notice a muscle you never had before. It may take three months before you see any progress at all, but once you do you'll see continual development. Then it's only a matter of time until you begin to notice some definition in your front thigh—a fine line being drawn down to give your leg a pretty look.

It may take a year before your thighs are perfect, but in six months everyone should see some major changes. We've heard reports of some women seeing results as early as six weeks, but these women are lucky. Don't worry if it takes you longer. Once you develop attractive thighs, they're yours to keep. They don't disappear. They're permanent—as long as you invest fifteen minutes three times a week to keep them toned and shapely, which should become easier and easier with time.

EXERCISES

There are five exercises for the thighs. If you are working at home, follow the home routine, which is given first in this chapter. If you're working in the gym, see pages 180–185 for your routine.

HOME THIGH ROUTINE

1. Leg curl with a weight
2. Front squat
3. Lunge with buttocks squeeze
4. Sissy squat
5. Bugs Bunny lunge

GYM THIGH ROUTINE

1. Leg curl
2. Front squat
3. Lunge with buttocks squeeze
4. Machine leg extension
5. Leg press

Do seven to eleven repetitions for each of your three exercise sets, using the same weight. Don't forget to raise your weight if you're getting more than eleven reps for each set.

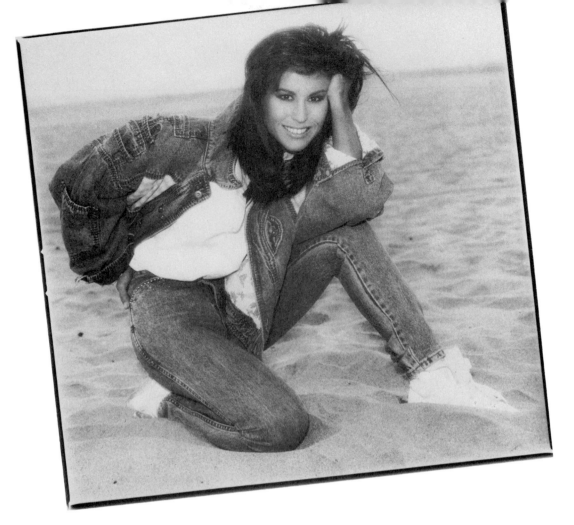

HOW OFTEN TO WORK OUT

You should work your thighs three times a week or every other day, unless you are working your whole body and doing the four-day split routine. Then it's okay to work them only twice a week. (See page 47 for details on the four-day split routine.)

WARM-UP/PRE-STRETCH

Stand in a natural position with your back erect. Lift your left leg behind you and grab your ankle with your left hand. Pull your leg as close to your buttocks as possible or until you feel the stretch in your thigh area. Hold the position for a count of ten and repeat for the other leg.

Now stand with your feet together and bend over slowly to stretch the hamstring muscles of your back thighs. Grasp your ankles to increase the stretch, and hold through a count of ten. Release and repeat.

Prior to performing each exercise, select a very light weight and do fifteen to twenty warm-up repetitions. Then start your regular sets. Remember, this light set does not count as one of your required three sets. If the exercise requires no weight, of course, you need not do a light warm-up set. Just begin your routine.

170 HOME THIGH ROUTINE

Leg Curl with a Weight

This leg curl perfects the biceps femoris—the back thigh, or hamstring, muscle.

POSITIONING

- Place a dumbbell between your feet and lie face down on a padded exercise bench.
- Place your knees about an inch or two over the edge of the bench.
- Hold the weight tightly with your feet.

THE MOVEMENT

- Bending at the knees, raise your lower legs until they are perpendicular to the floor.
- Flex (squeeze) your biceps femoris, then return to start position.
- Repeat the movement until you have completed your set.

REMEMBER

- Never jerk the weight up. Control it and concentrate on your back thigh muscles.
- Never let the weight just pull you back down to start position. The down movement is just as important as the up. Keep your mind on the back of your thighs.
- Resist the temptation to raise your abdomen from the bench. Remain flat on the bench throughout the movement or you will remove some of the necessary stress from your back thigh muscles.

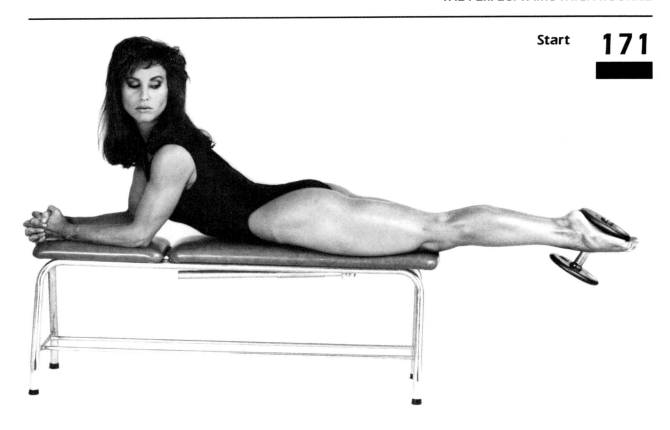

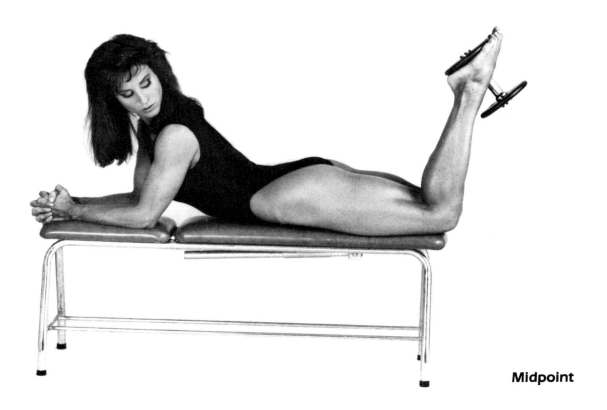

Midpoint

172 Front Squat

Front squats perfect both the quadriceps (front thigh muscle) and the buttocks. They are best done while looking into a mirror to help maintain perfect form.

POSITIONING

■ Place a barbell on a squat rack, lower your body under the bar, then lift it onto your upper chest–shoulder area.
■ Hold the bar with your palms facing upward and take a grip that is slightly wider than your shoulder width.
■ Angle your toes slightly outward (a natural position), and plant your feet firmly on the ground.

THE MOVEMENT

■ Keeping your upper body erect, slowly bend at the knees and lower your body until you are in a squat position. Your buttocks should be slightly lower than your knees. Feel the stretch in your quadriceps (front thighs).
■ Return to start position, controlling the weight, and flex (squeeze) your quadriceps muscle.
■ Repeat the movement until you have completed your set.

REMEMBER

■ Balance is essential. If you feel off balance, try the movement with a two-by-four board under your heels.
■ Always flex on the up movement and feel the stretch on the down movement. Keep your mind on your front thigh muscles throughout the exercise.
■ Be careful not to simply let yourself drop to the low position and never spring up to start. Keep your quadriceps working fluidly at all times.
■ Protect your knees by mentally telling your quadriceps to do the work. Picture only that muscle working. Tell your knees not to get too involved. Use your mind. Concentration is 99 percent of control.

Start

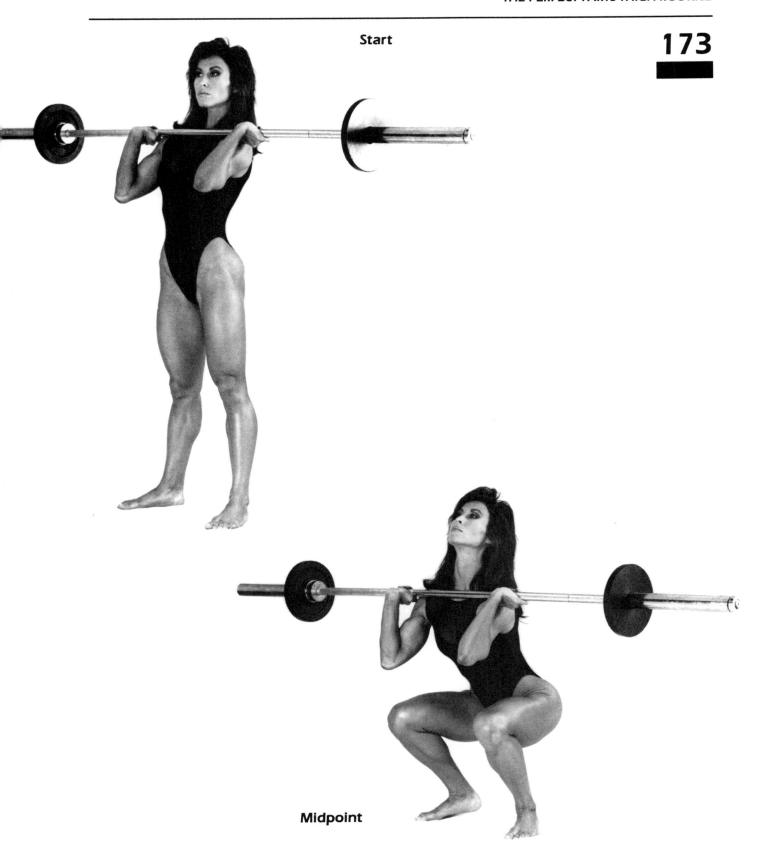

Midpoint

174   **Start**

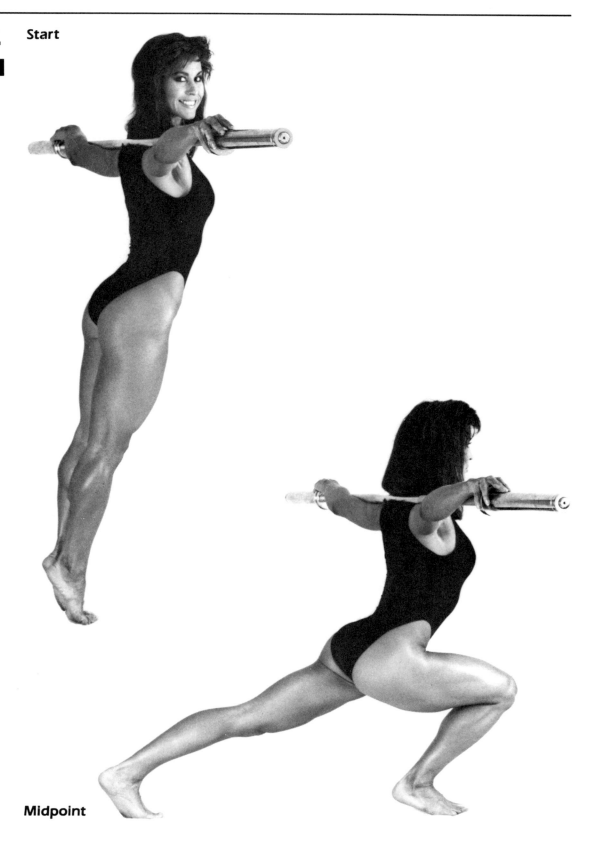

Midpoint

Lunge

Lunges perfect the front thigh (quadriceps) muscle, the hip muscles, and the buttocks. You may also do the buttocks squeeze lunge variation described in the preceding chapter.

POSITIONING

- Place a barbell across your shoulders and let it rest on your trapezius muscle.
- Hold the barbell in a wide grip that is comfortable to you. (I like to hold the bar right near the plates at either end.)
- Place your feet shoulder width apart, and point your toes straight ahead.

THE MOVEMENT

- Keeping your left leg straight, step forward with your right foot about two to three feet.
- Bend your right knee and "lunge" forward as far as you can. Feel the stretch in your quadriceps.
- Look straight ahead in the direction of movement in order to keep yourself from losing balance and leaning forward.
- Return to start position without bouncing, and repeat the movement until you have completed your set.

REMEMBER

- It takes time to feel comfortable with this exercise. Don't despair if you feel awkward and occasionally lose your balance during the first few weeks.
- Don't bounce harshly off your leg when rising to the up position. Remain in total control, and keep your mind on your front thigh muscle.

176 Sissy Squat

This exercise perfects the quadriceps (front thigh) muscle. Do this exercise *immediately* after you complete your lunges.

POSITIONING

- Stand in front of a stable post or bar and grip it for balance.
- Place your feet shoulder width apart.
- Stand at arms' length from the post, with your arms stretched out completely in front of you and your toes pointed out.

THE MOVEMENT

- Raise yourself up on your toes and lean your upper body back to a 45-degree angle with the floor while bending your legs to a right angle and thrusting your knees and hips as far forward as possible. (Your hips should be in line with your ankles.)
- Feel the complete stretch in your quadriceps muscles as you lower your body.
- Return to start position and repeat the movement without resting until you have completed your set.

REMEMBER

- You must do this exercise in strict form in order to gain the benefit. Look at the pictures and read the instructions. Soon it will become easy.
- Since you use no weight for this exercise, do fifteen strict repetitions for each set.
- Realize that this is not an exercise to build size, but an exercise to stretch and shape the thigh. It is a must for gorgeous thighs.

Start

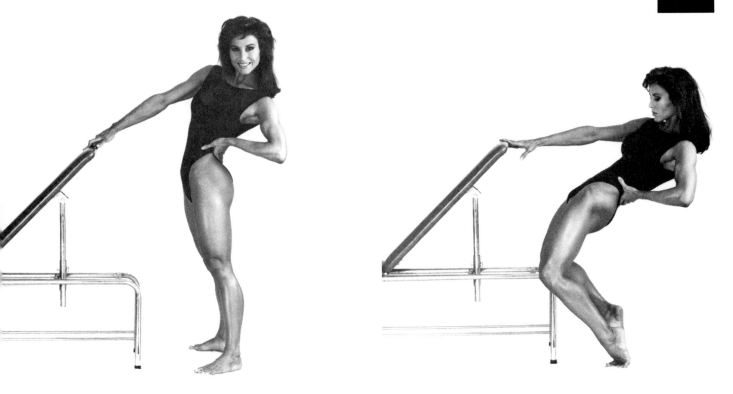

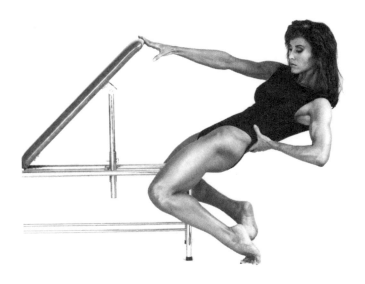

178   **Start**

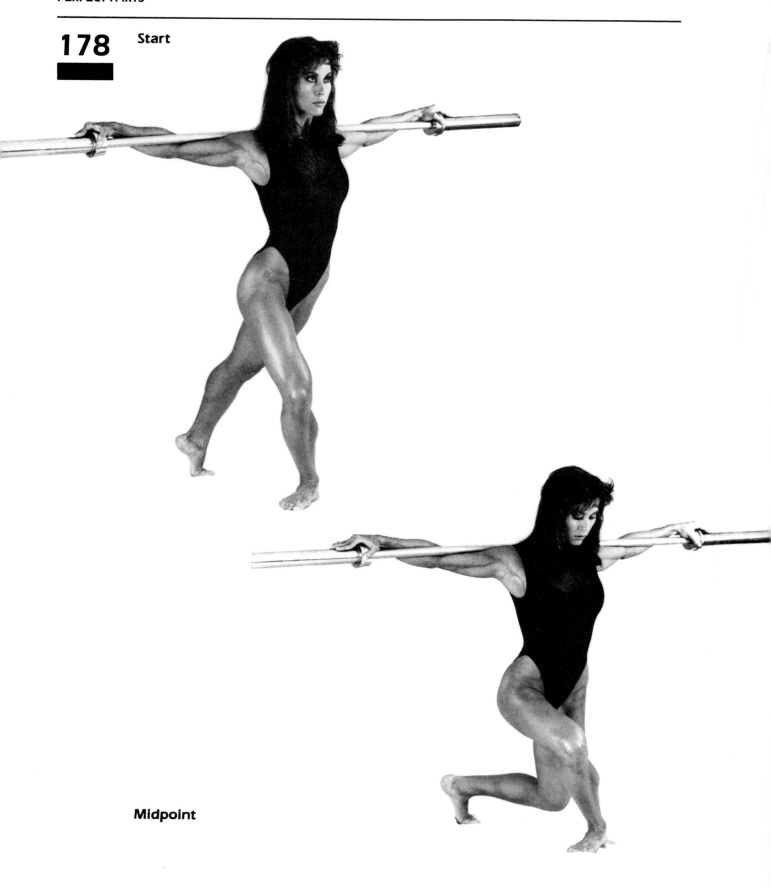

Midpoint

Bugs Bunny Lunge

Bugs Bunny lunges perfect the inner thigh, buttocks, and upper back thigh.

POSITIONING

- Place a barbell on your shoulders, letting it rest on your trapezius muscles.
- Standing erect, extend your right foot in front of you, pointing your toes outward.
- Stand on your toes on your left foot, pointing the toes on that foot outward also.

THE MOVEMENT

- Lunge forward by bending both knees until the left knee is about three inches off the ground.
- Straighten your legs and return to the start position, feeling the flex in your inner thighs and buttocks, and repeat the movement twice on the same side.
- Reverse leg positions and repeat the movement in the same way three times.
- Alternate legs until you have completed your set.
- Use the principle of muscle contraction specificity to affect development of the inner thighs.

REMEMBER

- Keep your mind on your quadriceps muscles at all times.
- Let your front thigh muscles stretch and flex with each movement.
- Take your time and learn to do the exercise correctly. It is unique and very effective.

180 GYM THIGH ROUTINE

Leg Curl

Leg curls perfect the biceps femoris—the back thigh, or hamstring, muscles.

POSITIONING

- Lie face down on the padded table of the leg curl machine.
- Place your heels under the roller pads and grasp the handles on either side of the table. (If no handles are provided, you can hold onto the sides of the table.)

THE MOVEMENT

- Bend your legs at the knees, raising your feet upward until your lower legs are perpendicular to the floor, with toes pointed up.
- Hold the position for a split second and return to start, controlling the weight as you lower your legs.
- Repeat the movement until you have completed your set.

REMEMBER

- Keep your mind on your biceps femoris (back thighs) throughout the exercise.
- Maintain control. Do not swing the weight up or simply let it pull your legs down.
- Concentrate on working hard and flexing on the up movement and stretching on the down movement.
- Keep your hips pressed against the table throughout the movement.

Front Squat

Follow the instructions on page 172.

Lunge

Follow the instructions on page 175.

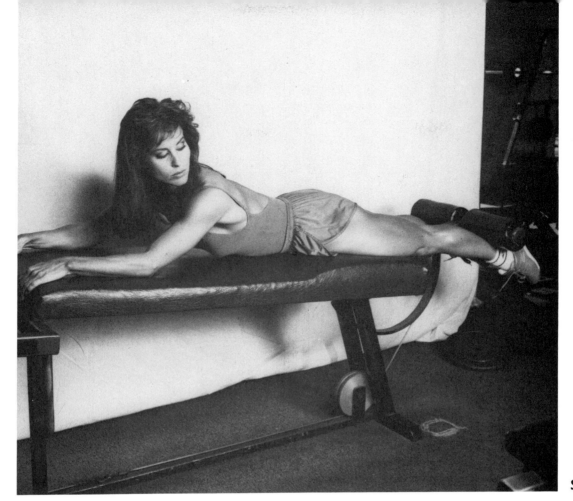

Start

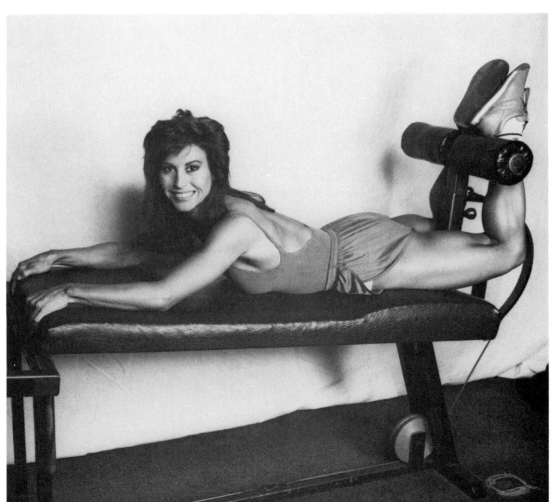

Midpoint

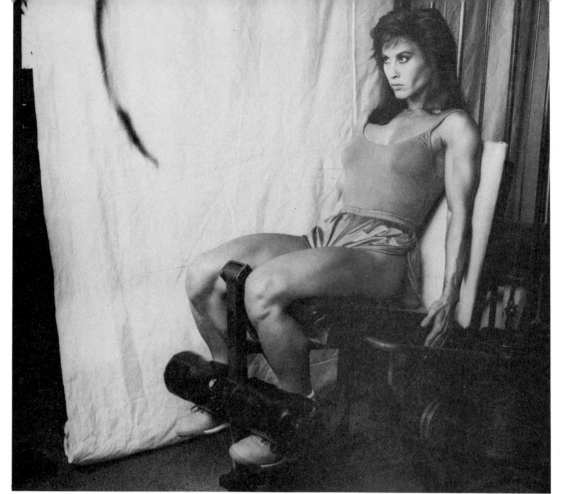

Start

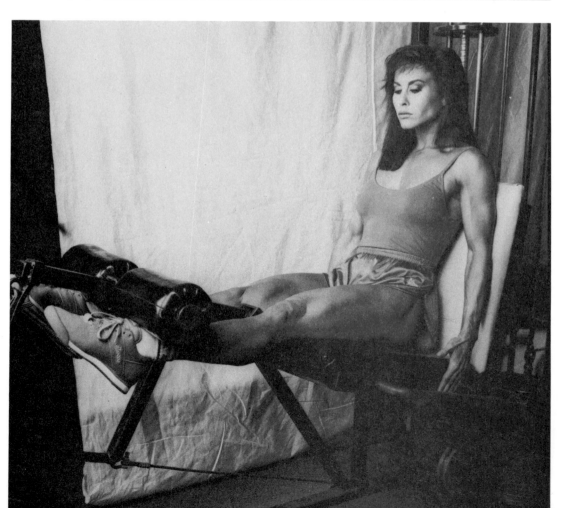

Midpoint

Leg Extension

This exercise perfects the quadriceps (front thigh) muscle.

POSITIONING

- Sit in the machine seat and place the top of your feet under the machine roller pad.
- Grasp the handles on the side of the seat on either side of you.

THE MOVEMENT

- Extend your legs until they are straight out in front of your body. Hold the position for a split second as you flex (squeeze) your quadriceps.
- Return to start in full control of the weight, and feel the stretch in your quadriceps.
- Repeat the movement until you have completed your set.

REMEMBER

- Be careful not to throw the weight up in a bouncing type of motion. Instead, raise it in full control, using only your quadriceps to do the work.
- Don't let the weight simply drop to the start position. Lower it slowly, using your quadriceps muscles.

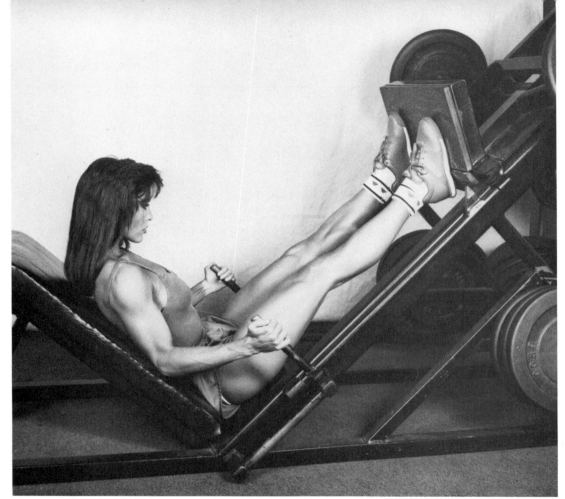

Start

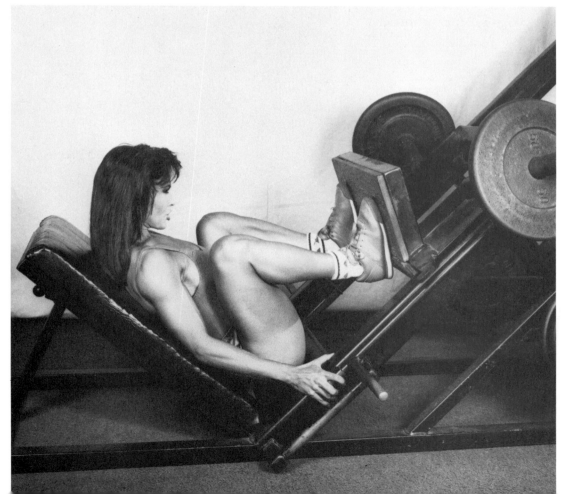

Midpoint

Leg Press

Leg presses perfect the quadriceps, the hip muscles, and the buttocks.

POSITIONING

■ There are several kinds of leg press machines. We will describe the movement for the standard leg press, in which you lie on your back and push the weight upward. You can easily adjust the instructions here to any other type of machine.

■ Lie flat on your back on the padded surface of the leg press machine, and release the weighted platform by turning the handles on either side of you.

■ Place your feet shoulder width apart against the foot surface of the machine, with your toes pointed very slightly outward. (This requires you to bend your knees sharply.)

■ Grasp the sides of the padded surface.

THE MOVEMENT

■ Push the weight platform up by extending your legs until your knees are almost completely locked, and flex (squeeze) your quadriceps muscles.

■ Maintaining full control, return to the start position.

■ Repeat the movement until you have completed your set.

REMEMBER

■ Be sure to feel the flex on the upward movement and the stretch on the downward movement.

■ Remain in control of the weight at all times. Raise it slowly, then lower it slowly, keeping your mind on your quadriceps muscle throughout the movement.

■ Never let your mind wander. Prevent injury by concentrating on what you're doing.

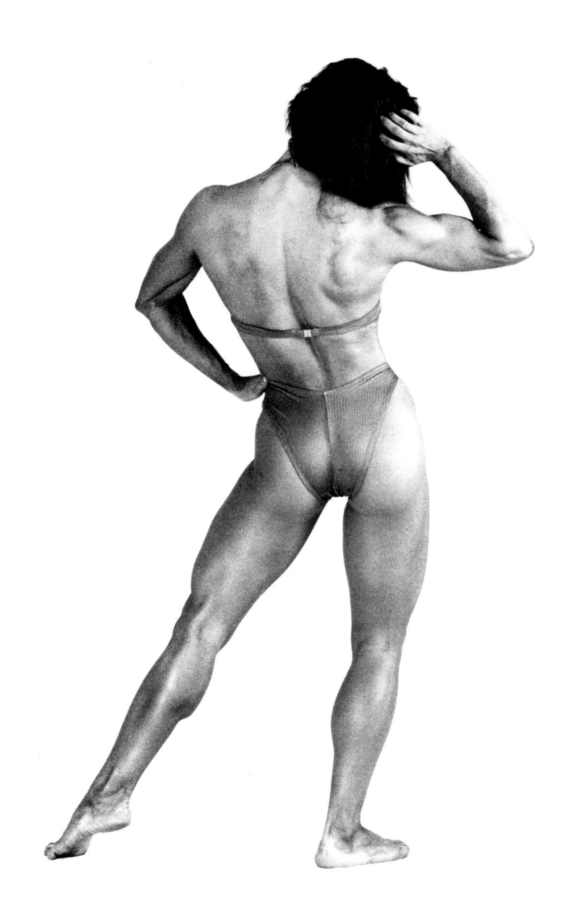

15

The <u>Perfect Parts</u> Calf Routine

Until recently, calf muscles were the only muscles women were always "allowed" to have without censure. Well-developed calves have traditionally been considered an asset to the feminine physique.

As far back as the Middle Ages, well-developed calves on a woman were considered a dangerous asset because of the undue temptation they presented males. As a result, women were required to wear their dresses floor length so that they would not unwittingly lure men into sin. It was not until the 1920s that fashion took the daring step of allowing this sensual part of a woman's body to be seen in public. But that made weak calves as visible as perfect calves.

If you have well-formed thighs and underdeveloped calves, your legs will look top heavy, no matter how perfectly formed your thigh is. In addition, your buttocks will seem larger, because a pencil-thin or flat calf throws attention upward to the roundness of the buttocks.

It's foolish to work hard to have a beautiful body and then neglect your calf muscle, which responds so readily to training and needs so few exercises in order to be perfected. So come on, you might as well go for the complete look.

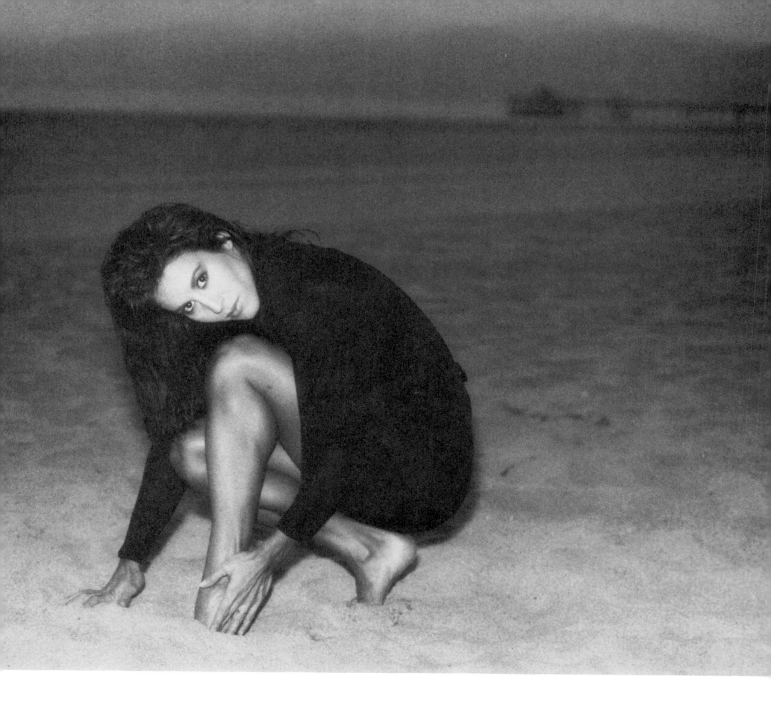

THE CALF MUSCLES

The calf muscle consists of two muscles, the gastrocnemius and the soleus. The gastrocnemius in turn consists of two parts, which connect in the middle of the lower leg and tie in with the Achilles tendon. The section where the two heads of the muscle tie in to each other forms the raised calf muscle. The gastrocnemius muscle works to flex the knee and the foot downward.

The soleus lies beneath the gastrocnemius, and it assists in flexing the foot downward.

DEVELOPMENT

The calf is one of the easiest muscles for a woman to develop. You will probably see it beginning to take shape in a month or two. Some women will see development even sooner.

EXERCISES

There are three exercises in your calf routine. If you are working at home, follow the home routine, which is given first. If you are working in a gym or fitness center, follow the gym routine, which is found on pages 196–199.

HOME CALF ROUTINE

1. One-legged calf raise
2. Calf raise—ankle rotated
3. Seated dumbbell calf raise

GYM CALF ROUTINE

1. One-legged calf raise
2. Seated calf raise
3. Standing calf machine raise

Do three sets of seven to eleven repetitions for each exercise. If you find that you can do more than eleven repetitions for each set, then it's time to raise the weight.

Incidentally, the calves can withstand relatively heavy weights, so don't be surprised to find yourself going quite high in weight after a few months.

HOW OFTEN TO WORK OUT

Work your calves three times a week or every other day, unless you are working your entire body and following the split routine, in which case you will be working your calves only twice a week. (See page 47 for a review of the split routine.)

WARM-UP/PRE-STRETCH

The best stretch for your calves is the favorite used by runners, the "Achilles stretch." Place your feet together and position yourself two and a half to three feet from a wall. Place your hands flat on the wall, leaning forward, arms extended fully. Keep your back straight and bend at the elbows and lower your body toward the wall until your elbows touch the wall. Keep your heels on the ground and your feet flat throughout the movement. Hold the position for a count of ten. Repeat the stretch two more times.

Do one set of fifteen to twenty repetitions of each exercise, using a light weight. This does not count as one of your regular sets, which will be done at regular weight with from seven to eleven repetitions.

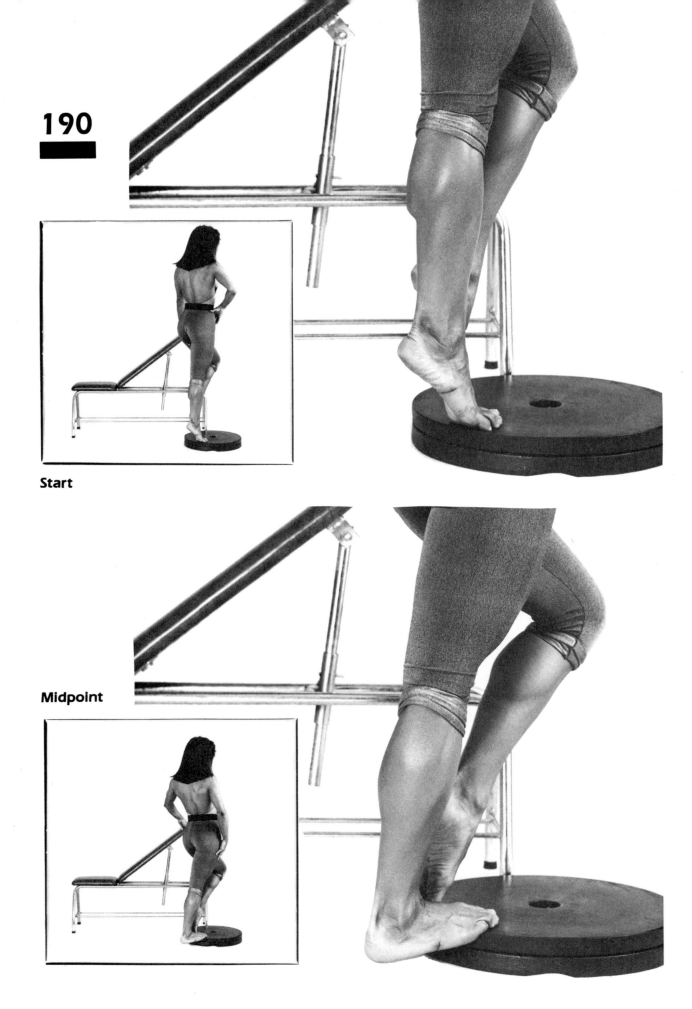

190

Start

Midpoint

HOME CALF ROUTINE

One-legged Calf Raise—Toes Forward

This exercise perfects the gastrocnemius muscle.

POSITIONING

- Place a block of wood on the floor near a holding device.
- Hold a dumbbell in your left hand and stand on the block of wood so that your heel and arch are completely off the block of wood. (The block must be high enough so that when you extend your heel downward, it does not touch the floor.)
- Hold onto the device and stand erect.
- Raise your right foot off the floor and out of the way.
- With the toes of your left foot pointing straight ahead, lower your left heel as low as possible.

THE MOVEMENT

- Raise yourself onto your left toes and feel the flex in your calf muscle.
- Lower yourself, again extending your heel down as far as possible, and feel the stretch in your calf muscle.
- Repeat the set for your other leg.
- Alternate sets until you have completed your exercise.

REMEMBER

- Do not bounce up and down. Use controlled movements and concentrate on your calf muscles.
- Remember to pyramid the weights. You should hold a heavier dumbbell for each set and do less reps (as described in chapter 6).

192

Start

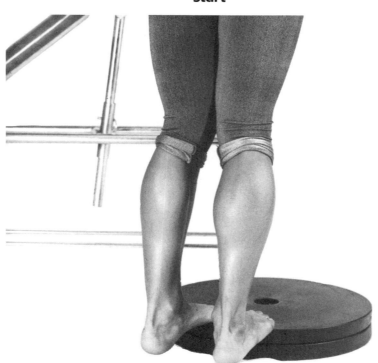

Midpoint

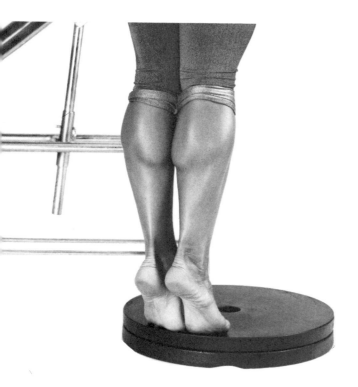

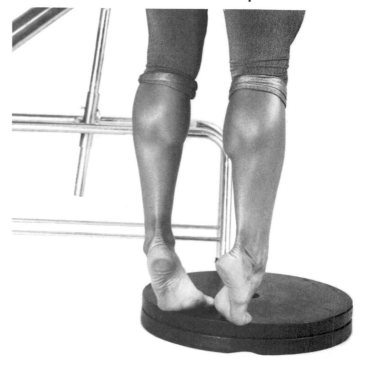

Calf Raise—Ankle Rotated

This exercise perfects the calves from all angles and strengthens the arches of your feet.

POSITIONING

■ Stand on a platform or ledge so that your weight is on the balls of your feet and your heels extend out over the edge.
■ With your feet close together, pigeon-toe style, lower your heels as far down as you can.

THE MOVEMENT

■ Lift up on your toes, simultaneously rotating your feet inward on the big toe area of the balls of your feet.
■ When you reach the highest point of your movement, slowly rotate your feet outward.
■ Lower your heels back to the start position.

REMEMBER

■ Strive for slow, deliberate contractions.
■ Concentrate on your calf muscles as you control the movement perfectly.

194 **Start**

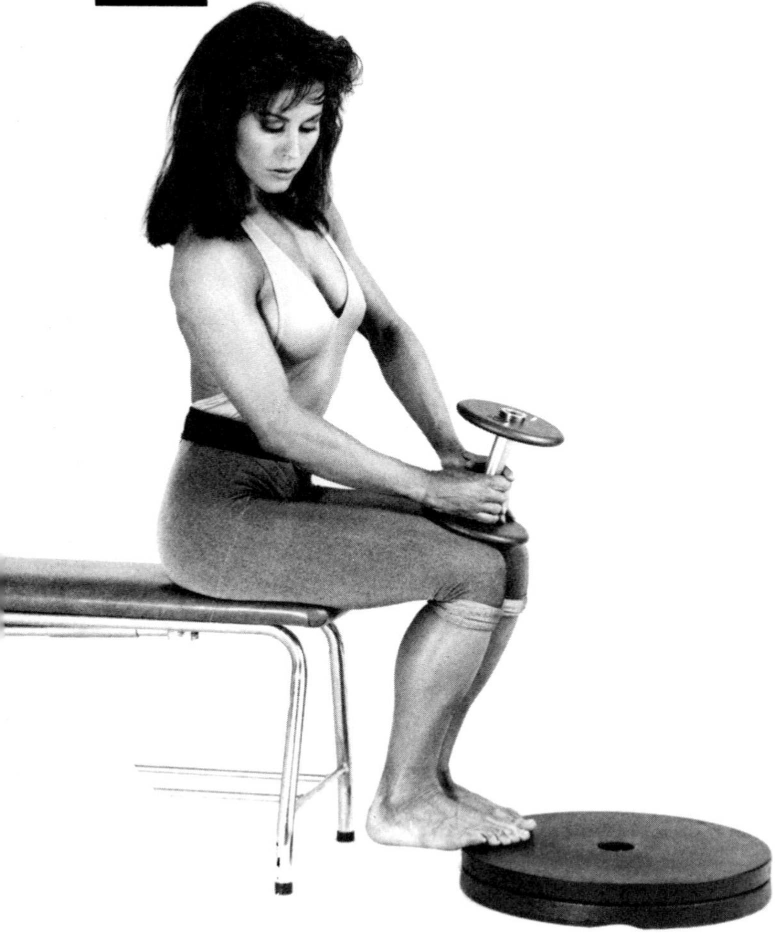

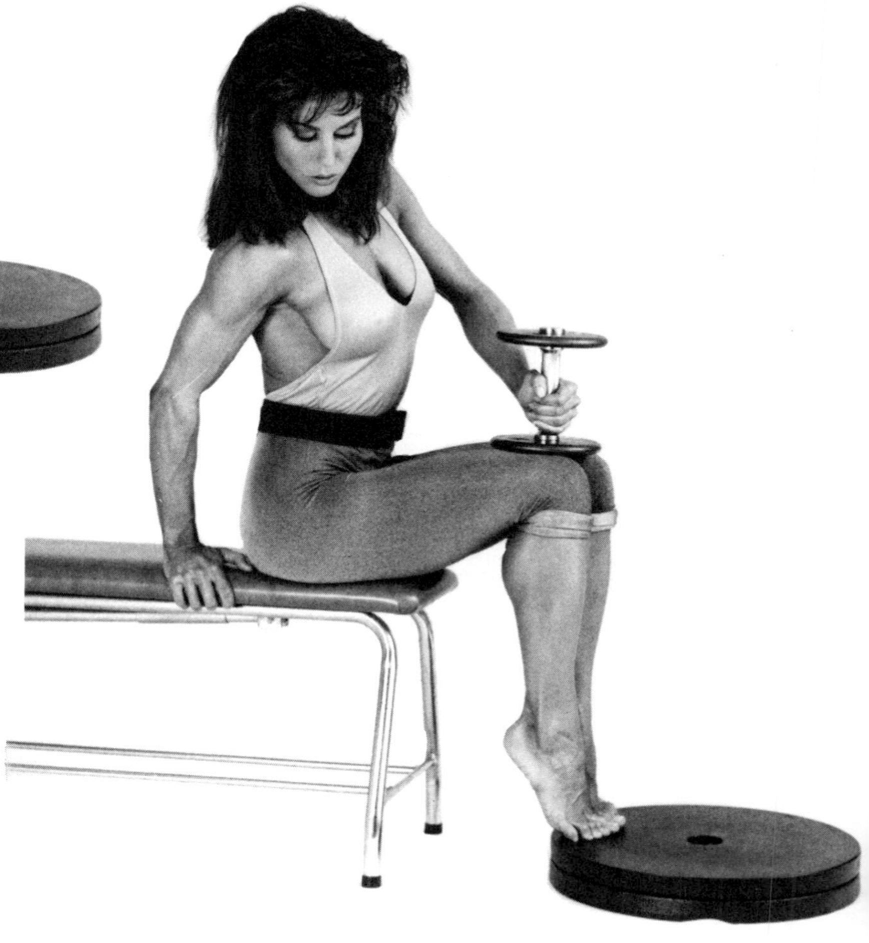

Midpoint

Seated Dumbbell Calf Raise

This exercise helps develop the gastrocnemius and especially the broad soleus muscles located just below the gastrocnemius.

POSITIONING

■ Sit on the edge of a flat bench or sturdy chair and position your legs in an L position.

■ Place a block of wood about five inches high under your toes, and stand on the edge of the wood so that your heels are off the wood and can extend downward for the exercise.

■ Place a dumbbell between your thighs, close to your knees, and hold it there.

■ Lower your heels as far down as possible.

THE MOVEMENT

■ Raise your toes as high as possible, and feel the flex in your calf muscles.

■ Lower your heels as far down as possible and feel the stretch in your calf muscle.

■ Repeat the movement until you have completed your set.

REMEMBER

■ Don't bounce the weight up and down. Keep your mind on your calf muscles and maintain a steady, even movement.

■ Remember to flex hard and to stretch completely with each up and down movement.

VARIATION

■ To get muscle contraction specificity, rotate your ankles as described in the preceding exercise.

196 GYM CALF ROUTINE

One-Legged Calf Raise

Follow instructions on page 191.

Seated Calf Raise

This exercise perfects the entire calf area.

POSITIONING

- Adjust the calf machine so that your knees fit comfortably under the padded knee rest.
- Place the soles of your feet on the metal foot bar, making sure that your heels are completely off the bar so that they can be fully extended downward for the exercise.
- Lower your heels to the lowest possible point.

THE MOVEMENT

- Raise your knees as high as possible, doing the work with your calves.
- Flex your calves on the highest position, then return to start, letting your calves stretch fully on the lowest position.
- Repeat the movement until you have completed your set.

REMEMBER

- Resist the temptation to rush through the exercise.
- Do not bounce on the up and down movement. Concentrate on working your calf muscles through maintaining perfect form and control.

197

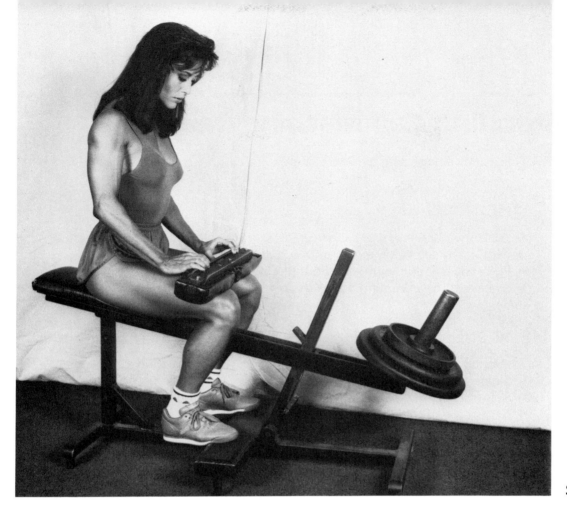

Start

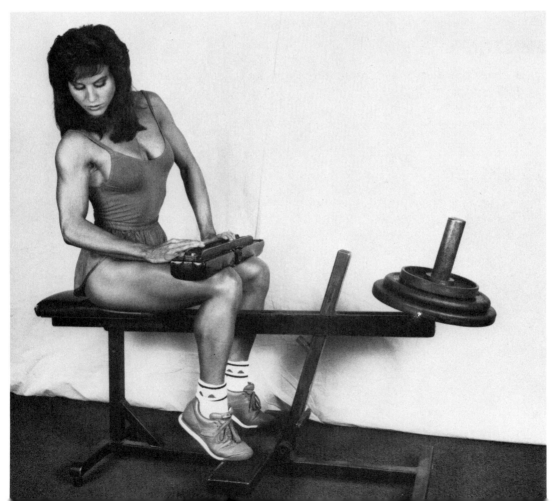

Midpoint

198 Standing Calf Machine Raise

This exercise perfects the entire calf area.

POSITIONING

- Position yourself in the calf machine by facing the machine and getting under the padded yoke.
- Place the soles of your feet about three inches apart on the bar provided, and let your heels descend as low as possible.

THE MOVEMENT

- Rise up on your toes as high as possible, doing the work with your calf muscles. Flex your calves on the highest point.
- Return to the start position, letting your calf muscles stretch fully.
- Repeat the movement until you have completed your set.

REMEMBER

- Avoid the temptation to bounce up and simply drop down. Control the weight at all times. Keep your mind on your calf muscles.

VARIATION

- To achieve muscle contraction specificity, rotate your ankles during the up movement.

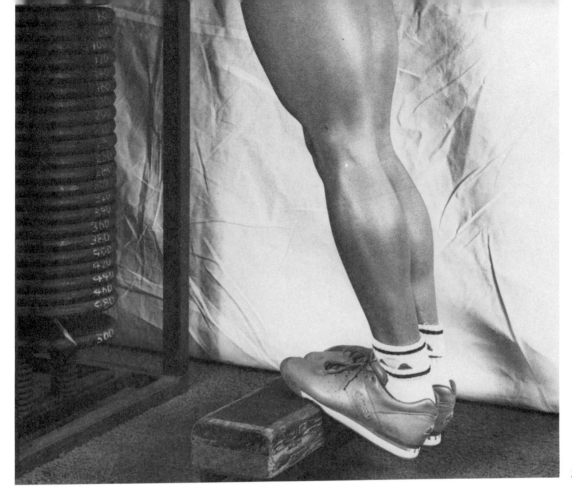

Start

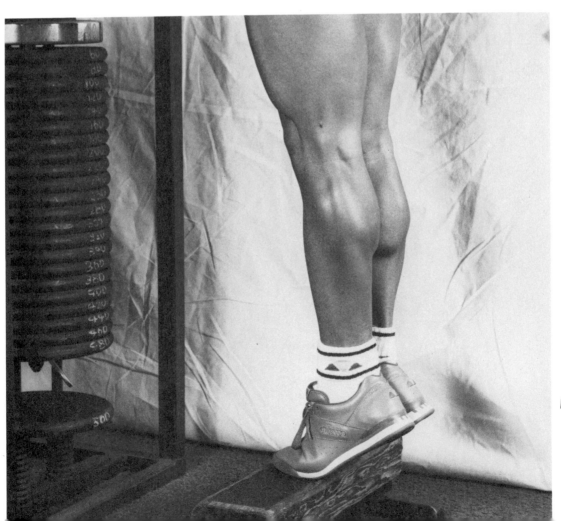

Midpoint

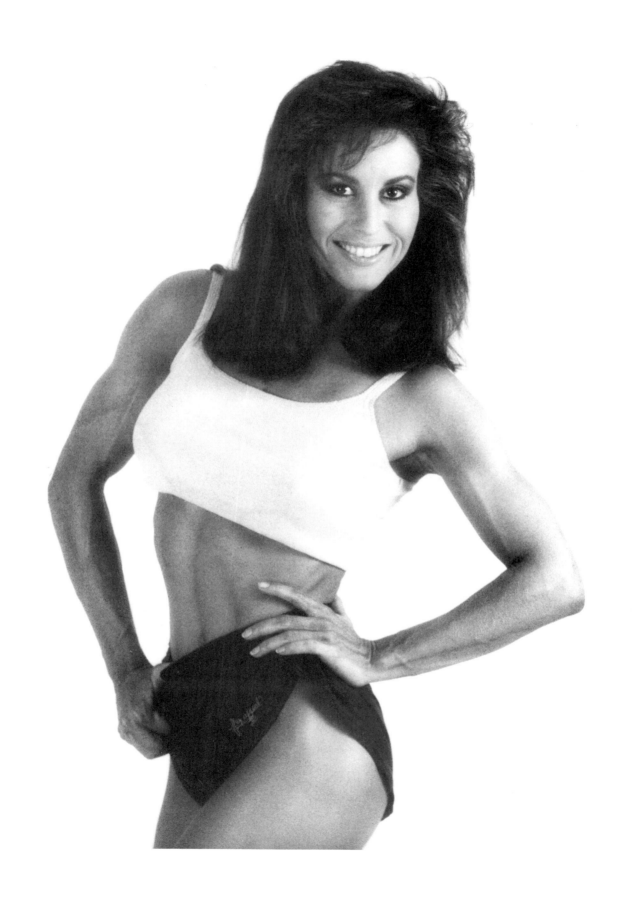

16

The Perfect Diet

There is no way around it. In order to see your perfectly formed muscles, you'll have to eliminate excess body fat. This is the fat that forms as a result of overeating. It forms right under your skin, and the result is to hide the shape of your muscles.

Note that I specified *excess* body fat. I want to make it clear that I am not encouraging a compulsive, obsessive approach to diet in which you continually starve yourself because you are never satisfied that you are thin enough. That leads to ill health. Taken to extremes, it can be life-threatening. Some body fat is natural—in fact, it is necessary to good health. But when there's a noticeable layer of flab to be seen in the mirror, it makes sense to look for a healthy way to be rid of it.

Compared to what you have to do to build muscles, getting rid of fat is easy. All you have to do is adjust your food intake. You don't have to starve; there's no reason ever to go hungry. (If you do find yourself going hungry, you can be sure you are eating the wrong way.)

Adjusting food intake requires two points of focus: (1) limiting quantities so that you don't consume more calories than you burn off daily—or, if you are on a reducing diet, so that you consume less calories than you burn off daily; (2) making sure you eat the right combination of foods to ensure getting the nutrients required to maintain good health—including when you are on a diet.

Good eating requires intelligence. There are foods that provide your body maximum energy and foods that provide the raw material for muscle-building. Some foods

201

take more energy to digest, which means fewer calories will be absorbed into your system. For example, it takes only 5 percent of the energy content of the fat you eat to convert to body fat, but it takes 20 percent of the energy content of the carbohydrates and protein you eat to convert to body fat.

So, a calorie is *not* a calorie is not a calorie. It isn't true that no matter what you eat, every 3500 calories will work the same in your system, with the same potential to be converted to fat. It does matter what you eat.

To put it simply, if you are at all overweight there's one thing you *don't* want to do—eat fat. You don't want to consume butter, mayonnaise, the skin of chicken or turkey, or fried foods, which have soaked up loads of fat. (Just because you can't see the fat, don't think it's not there.) You don't want to eat meat that is loaded with fat.

There's more than vanity involved. Besides hiding your "good looks potential," the body fat you develop as a result of poor eating habits can adversely affect your health. It can lead to hypertension, heart trouble, diabetes, senility—and premature death.

Before I give you a delicious weight loss diet and a surprisingly enjoyable maintenance diet that will allow you to eat anything you please one day a week, let's talk about what is and what is not good for your lovely body. You should understand the basic facts about calories and food content, and you should learn which foods are good for you and which foods are energy drainers/fat gainers and hence enemies. The best appetite suppressant is a well-nourished body.

WHAT IS A CALORIE?

A calorie is a unit of energy supplied to your body by the food you eat. There are 4 calories in every gram of protein and 4 calories in every gram of carbohydrate, but there are 9 calories in every gram of fat.

Everyone needs a minimum calorie intake in order to stay alive. You probably need between 1800 and 2500 calories just to maintain your present body weight *even if you are not overweight.*

The kinds of calories you consume are important because they affect your energy level.

CARBOHYDRATES ARE YOUR ENERGY AND BRAIN FOOD

When you eat carbohydrates your digestive system goes to work breaking them down into glucose, which your body and brain then use for energy. Without a sufficient amount of glucose supplied by carbohydrates, your energy level drops, your mind becomes unable to concentrate, and you become irritable. It becomes difficult for you to perform your daily chores without a great deal of effort—even getting up from a chair becomes a major project. Those of you who have tried the high-protein, low-carbohydrate diets know what I am talking about.

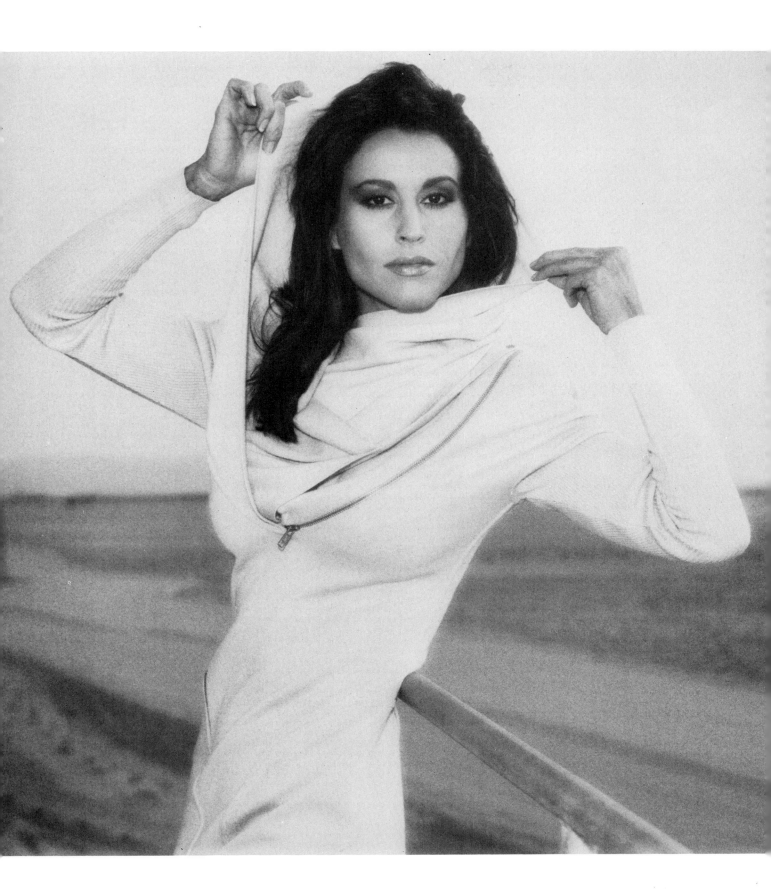

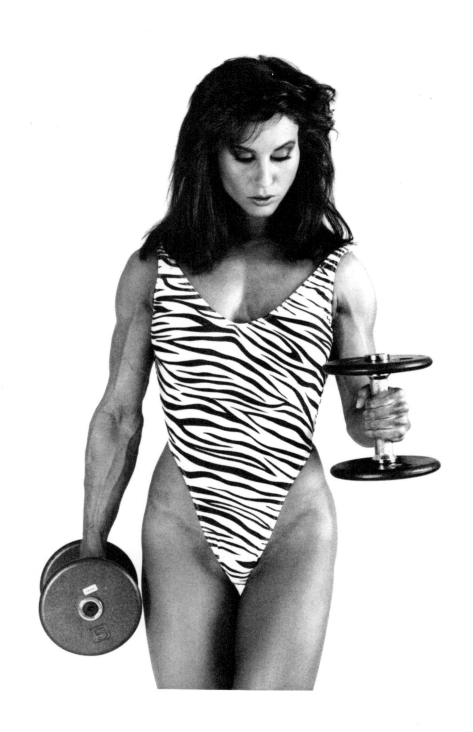

PROTEINS ARE YOUR BODY BUILDING FOOD

The basic building material of your body is protein. Your blood, skin, hair, nails, internal organs (even your heart and your brain), and all of your muscles are comprised mainly of protein. Dietary protein also helps your body to produce the hormones that control your metabolism.

However, protein is not a preferred energy source for your body. It is only when you deprive your body of the carbohydrates needed to satisfy its energy demands that your body becomes desperate enough to call upon protein for energy use. If you foolishly go on a very low carbohydrate diet, your body would not only use the energy of dietary protein calories to function, it would begin to burn actual muscle protein to use as energy. Instead of building muscle with your workout, you would lose muscle. Your goal is to lose fat, not muscle, so even when dieting keep your carbohydrates relatively high and your protein at a reasonable amount. (We'll discuss proportions later.)

FAT: FRIEND AND ENEMY

Your body needs some fat in order to function perfectly—but not nearly as much as most people consume. You should be consuming no more than 20 percent of your total daily calorie or energy consumption in fat. Most people consume from 30 to 50 percent of their daily calories in fat. Why? It is my guess that they do not realize where the fat is hidden. I will help you to discover where the fat is and teach you how to avoid it.

Fat is needed by the body to cushion the internal organs, the muscles, and the bones. It is also necessary for the proper absorption of vitamins A, E, K, and D, and the mineral calcium.

But you don't have to make an extra effort to ensure getting enough fat in your diet. You'll automatically get what you need in attending to your protein needs. There is fat in chicken, turkey, fish, eggs, milk, and cheese. In fact, you should choose the lowest fat content products possible when selecting protein foods, because you will still get more than the minimum amount needed. There is no need ever to go out of your way to eat fat in order to fulfill your basic fat requirement.

I'm not saying, however, that you can never eat an ice-cream cone or have a bagel and cream cheese again. Of course you can. Just realize that when you do, you are enjoying a treat that is not the most efficient and nutritious food for your body. But that's okay occasionally. What a bore it would be never again to be able to indulge in these foods. On the contrary, I encourage you to live it up once a week and eat whatever you please, *once you have lost your excess fat and are on the maintenance diet.*

206 CHOLESTEROL IS NOT ALL BAD

Cholesterol is a component of certain fats—primarily animal fats that are solid in form and "saturated," as opposed to the liquid, "unsaturated" fats that comprise vegetable, seed, nut, and grain oils. Cholesterol is present in meat, milk, milk products, and eggs. We all know that it can contribute to arteriosclerosis and heart attacks, but what most of us *don't* know is that cholesterol is essential to our health. It is the cholesterol in the skin that is converted to vitamin D through the action of the sun's ultraviolet rays. Cholesterol is also essential in the process of digesting carbohydrates, and it is cholesterol that supplies the body with natural adrenal steroid compounds such as cortisone and the sex hormones. It's not cholesterol per se that's a dietary problem. It's an excess of it that's a problem, that contributes to health difficulties.

If you are concerned that your cholesterol level is too high, don't worry and wonder. See your doctor and get a cholesterol count. If it is too high, he will suggest ways to lower it, which will include making dietary changes. Some foods are known to help lower cholesterol levels: eggplant, onion, garlic, yogurt, unpeeled apple, soybeans, carrots, and pinto, navy, and kidney beans.

If you have a high cholesterol level, you should also avoid smoking cigarettes, food additives such as BHT, caffeinated coffee, refined sugar, saturated fats.

Eggs have been blamed for causing high blood cholesterol levels, but recent research has vindicated the egg as an excellent source of nourishment. Eggs have the most perfect protein balance of any food, and they contain lecithin, which actually helps you emulsify (digest) fat. Eggs also help to raise your HDL (high density lipoprotein) level. HDL helps to break up cholesterol deposits, carrying it away from blood vessel walls to the liver for excretion. In effect, the higher your HDL level, the lower your chance of developing the symptoms of heart disease.*

VITAMINS AND MINERALS

Vitamins are organic substances found in foods. They are necessary for good health and life itself. Minerals are nutrients found in organic and inorganic combinations in foods and are necessary for the health of bones, all body organs, and the nervous system.

If you eat plenty of leafy greens, other dark green and yellow vegetables, and include some organ meats and whole grains in your regular diet, you will never have to worry about a deficiency of vitamins or minerals in your diet. If you are concerned about vitamin and mineral balance and feel you want to take vitamin or mineral supplements, I recommend you do so only under the supervision of your doctor or a qualified nutritionist. It is always better to get your vitamins and minerals the natural way—from real food. Think more than twice before you take any pill, even if it is a vitamin pill.

* See *Earl Mindell's New and Revised Vitamin Bible* by Earl Mindell (New York: Warner Books Inc., 1985, pp. 139–141) and *Heartplan: A Complete Guide for Total Fitness of Heart and Mind* by David Copen, M.D., and Mark Rubinstein, M.D. (New York: McGraw-Hill Book Co. Inc., 1987, pp. 18–19).

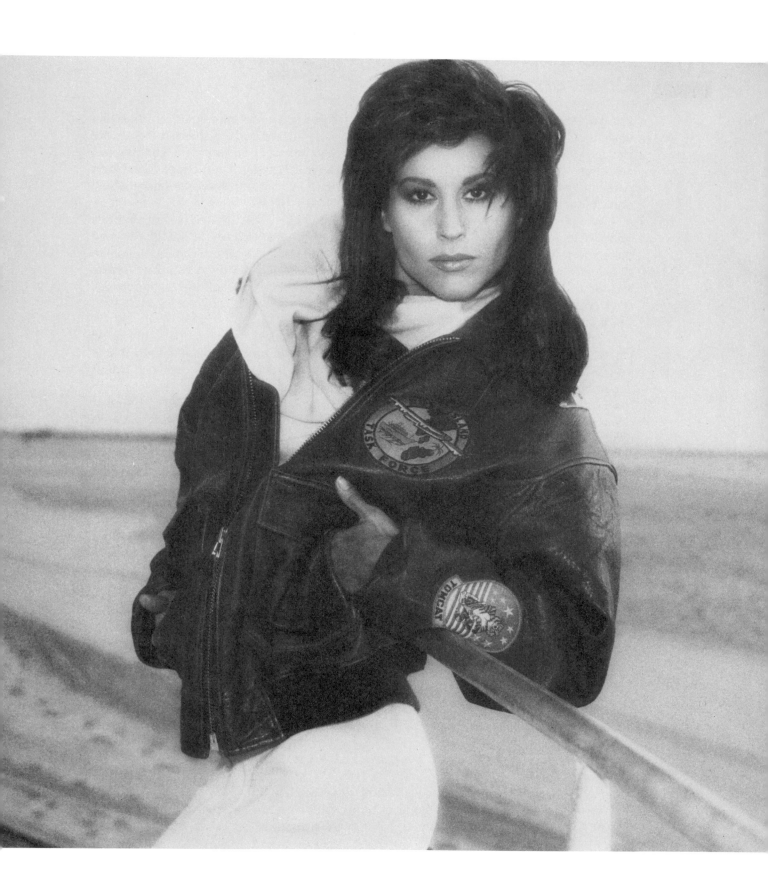

208 Special Minerals: Calcium and Sodium— Underdone and Overdone

I pair these two because most people lack a sufficient amount of calcium in their diet while they suffer from an overabundance of sodium. While both of these minerals are vital to good health, the right amount of them is even more important. Too little calcium can cause shrinking and weakened bones, and too much sodium can cause high blood pressure (which puts you at risk for stroke and heart attack) and water retention (which contributes to bloat that looks exactly like an ugly layer of fat).

Working out with weights helps to thicken and strengthen bones, so any worries about osteoporosis (the weakening and thinning of the bones) can be greatly reduced once you start this program. However, you need to support that with an adequate intake of calcium, so it's a good idea to include some high-calcium foods in your diet. These include all leafy green vegetables, broccoli, milk and milk products (low-fat, of course), nuts, and sardines (with bones). If you're in the mood for sweets, why not try molasses. It's high in calories but at least it's also high in calcium.

Sodium, most commonly taken in as salt (sodium chloride), is a hidden enemy. All canned foods are very high in sodium, and so are smoked foods. Chinese food that is prepared with MSG is also a culprit. Stay away from frozen dinners (but not frozen vegetables), fast-food hamburgers, pickles, and most sandwich meats. Start to read food labels, and get yourself a nutrition guide that indicates the sodium content of different foods. (See bibliography.) You'll be surprised to find how many high-sodium foods there are.

Any mention of sodium in a prepared food should be read as a warning to avoid or sharply limit your intake of that food. There is plenty of sodium in natural food. You don't need to go out of your way to find it. For example, one cup of broccoli, a recommended diet food, contains 450 milligrams of sodium. Get your sodium from fresh, nutritious foods, don't overdose on the salt added in canning. Most canned vegetables contain an added 1000 milligrams of sodium besides what is in the food itself. You don't need more than 2000 to 3000 milligrams for the entire day, so if you waste your sodium allotment on canned foods, you are sure to go over your allotment and pay the price of water retention and ugly bloat that looks just like fat.

WATER

You need lots of water. Drink at least eight glasses of water (distilled, if possible) a day, because it is only by drinking water that the inner body is bathed and cleansed. Water flushes lingering toxins out of your system. It also helps to moisturize your skin and curb your appetite.

Some people are under the false impression that the more water you drink, the more you will retain. Actually, the opposite is true. The more water you drink, the more cleansed your inner body and the less water you will retain.

You should really take advantage of times when you are naturally thirsty. Between sets of a good strong tennis match, I'll put away a glass or two of water, then I'll play again and really sweat it out. The more I sweat, the better I feel, because my body is being cleansed from the inside out.

WHAT IS A HEALTHY DIET?

A healthy diet is a balanced diet. Equally important, it is a diet you can live with on a day-to-day basis. You should never have to "go on a diet" in the sense that we commonly mean that. It is unnatural. What you should do is develop proper dietary habits that will satisfy your body and cause it to stop craving food poisons—substances such as processed sugars, saturated fats, and excessive sodium, all of which hinder our achieving the healthy vitality we seek.

Two-thirds of your daily food consumption should be in the form of carbohydrates. About 70 percent of the balance should be protein, and 30 percent fat.

SUGGESTED CARBOHYDRATE SOURCES FOR A BALANCED DIET

Carbohydrates come in two forms: simple and complex. Simple carbohydrates (notably refined and natural sugars) yield immediate energy; complex carbohydrates (notably whole grains and vegetables) release energy gradually. Avoid all processed simple carbohydrates, particularly foods containing refined sugar (candies, cookies, cakes, etc.), because although these give you a quick energy boost, that is followed by an even quicker let-down and a craving for an immediate refill. The end result is extra calories and less energy, which is not at all your goal. Stay with the nutritious simple carbohydrates, fruits.

Any fruit is fair game. You can delight your taste buds and at the same time get a quick shot of energy. But don't get into a rut and eat the same old fruits all the time. Go into your local fruit store and select a variety of fruits you've never eaten before. You'll be surprised to see that there are so many. Just walk around and when you see something different, ask the clerk what it is. Then buy it and try it. If you're curious to know how many calories it has, look it up in the *Nutrition Almanac* (see bibliography). Experiment. Have fun. You don't have to worry. Most fruits are not over 100 calories a piece. The only fruits to be wary of are avocados, which are high in saturated fats. (This is also true of coconuts.)

The best sources of gradually released energy are fresh and frozen vegetables. This includes the wonderful potato, which is so satisfying that it's hard to believe it contains only 100 calories. One potato takes care of: 33 percent of your daily vitamin C needs, 13 percent of your daily niacin needs, 10 percent of your daily thiamine needs, 8 percent of your daily phosphorus needs, and, believe it or not, 10 percent of your daily protein needs.

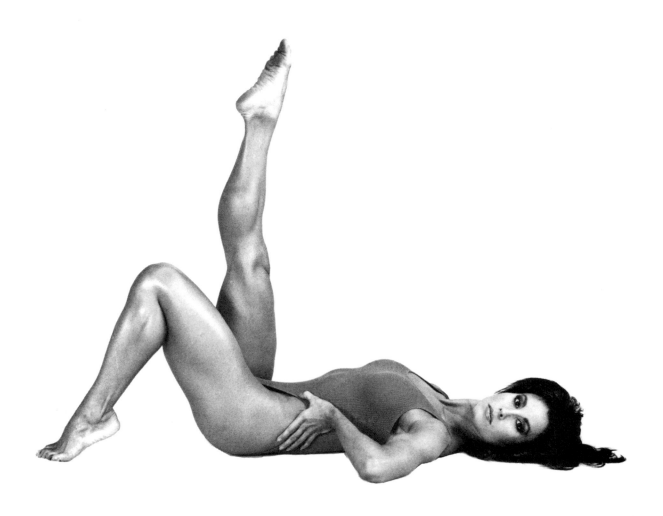

Other legitimate and deliciously satisfying sources of protein are pasta (especially high-protein or whole-wheat semolina), rice (brown or white), and whole-wheat and high-protein breads and cereals. Oatmeal is a frequently neglected but satisfying source of gradually released energy.

PROTEIN SOURCES FOR A BALANCED DIET

Although you can satisfy your protein needs by combining certain vegetable foods, unless you are a vegetarian, we suggest you stick to the best protein sources, which are white meat chicken and turkey, fish, lean beef, eggs (especially egg whites), and non-fat milk and milk products. If you are watching your calories, select low-calorie fish such as flounder, sole, or tuna, and eliminate the beef.

If you are a vegetarian, you can combine rice and soy beans, sprouted seeds, grains, and milk to meet your protein requirement. Fresh, raw vegetable juices also have lots of hidden protein.

THE <u>PERFECT PARTS</u> RAPID WEIGHT-LOSS DIET   211

If you follow this diet for a solid month, you will lose about 2 pounds a week, averaged out. In a month you will have lost between 8 and 10 pounds, but you will not feel deprived while you are dieting, and your body will not rebel and try to force you back into overeating once the diet is over. You will find it smooth sailing to go on the maintenance plan.

If you have more than 10 pounds to lose, you can either continue the one-month diet for another month or two or take a break from dieting by going on the maintenance plan for two weeks and then returning to the rapid weight-loss diet.

Rapid weight loss? You may be wondering how I can have the nerve to call a 2-pound-a-week weight loss rapid. Well, it is. Two pounds is the very maximum of fat that your body can lose in a week. Any other weight loss you register on the scale is really only a loss of water weight. We're not counting that. For example, in any given week that you are on this diet, the scale may show a 5- or even 7-pound loss. Don't get too excited. Included in that is water loss. In the long run, you will average out 2 pounds of *fat loss* a week, and that is fantastic! If your body weight drops more than 10 pounds in thirty days, then you are losing water because you have lowered the salt in your diet. That's good. You are getting a bonus. Water bloats you and it weighs you down. But permanent fat loss comes no faster than about 2 pounds a week, so be patient.

In starting this diet, make up your mind right now to drink lots of water. I want you to drink a glass of water before and after every meal, and a glass of water upon waking and going to bed. Period. No negotiations. Water is vital to your health and *it curbs your appetite.* And don't worry about adding water weight. That's not a function of how much you drink, that's a result of how much you *retain* as a result of poor mineral balance in the average diet and hence in your body.

You can make the water more interesting by heating it up and putting lemon juice in it, or adding a squeezed lemon or a tablespoon of orange juice to cold water.

Now, this is what you will eat, every day, for a month.

Breakfast

1 egg yolk and 4 egg whites, poached or scrambled *without* oil or butter
1 slice of whole-wheat toast, no butter

You can replace the eggs with 6 ounces of low-fat cottage cheese or 6 ounces of hoop cheese any day you wish, or substitute 6 ounces of low-fat yogurt and a piece of fresh fruit.

Snack

Two hours after breakast, eat any fruit (except avocado)—one only. It can be large.

212

Lunch

1 to 3 cups of steamed vegetables (choose a variety)
1 or 2 medium chicken breasts, broiled without the skin

One of the vegetables you choose should always be a green, leafy vegetable.

You can replace the chicken breasts with 6 ounces of water-packed tuna, but drain and rinse it to eliminate excess sodium. You can use vinegar, lemon, all sorts of spices, or no-oil salad dressing on the tuna.

Snack

Two hours after lunch, eat one fruit (any kind except avocado), ten raw almonds, or one cup freshly extracted vegetable juice.

Dinner

1 to 3 cups of steamed vegetables
Lettuce and tomato salad
1 or 2 medium chicken breasts or 6 ounces low-fat fish

You can substitute a baked or boiled potato for one of the cups of steamed vegetables.

You can substitute 6 ounces of white-meat turkey for the chicken. If you decide on fish, select from among flounder, sole, red snapper, or tuna (water-packed if canned; rinse and drain before eating).

Evening Snack

Have one piece of fruit, one cup freshly extracted vegetable juice, or a baked potato and as much lettuce (seasoned with vinegar), celery sticks, radishes, or sliced cucumber as you desire. You can also have a no-calorie soft drink if you desire, but I don't recommend this for every day. Do not eat any food after 8:00 P.M.

Beverages

You can have up to two cups of regular coffee a day if you so choose. Be aware that colas, even diet colas, have caffeine and lots of other chemicals, so avoid colas. Drink seltzer water—the new flavored ones are great—and have herbal teas. You can put low-fat milk in your coffee or tea if you wish. Freshly extracted vegetable juices are always great for you.

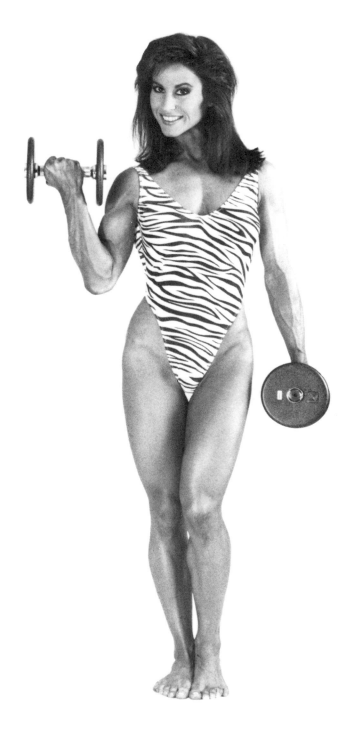

Diet Variations

Twice a week, you can have 4 ounces of pasta with low-fat marinara sauce in place of one of the cups of vegetables, or one cup of rice spiced any way you choose or with low-sodium tomatoes or tomato juice heated to a sauce.

214

WHAT IF YOU BLOW THE DIET?

Don't make the mistake of thinking, "Oh well, I had this cookie, I might as well eat half a pizza." I know you will slip once in a while. Just realize your mistake and resolve to use more self-control next time. You'll still lose a lot of fat weight, even if you make little mistakes every so often. You're learning something new—positive self-control in eating, and any new learning process involves falling and getting up again. Expect to succeed and if you make mistakes don't be too hard on yourself. I think you're going to make it. The fact that you're reading this book shows you mean business.

CHANGE YOUR MENTALITY

I don't want you to think about food all the time. That's why I don't make a big deal about your snacking any time during the day on luscious fresh vegetables. But I don't want to provide an extensive list of "free" eating snacks, or I would be teaching you that food is the main concern in life. It isn't. Food is a part of life. It's necessary to eat and it's fun to eat, but food is not life. It's only a part of life and it should be kept in perspective.

Learn to readjust your thinking about food. (Joyce's book *Now or Never*—see the bibliography that follows—has a complete discussion of how to use your subconscious mind to change your eating habits.) Start going out for dinner in restaurants with friends, even when you are on this diet. You can virtually always get broiled fish or chicken and steamed vegetables in a restaurant. Learn to enjoy the ambiance and the atmosphere. Don't hide from the world just because you are on a diet. But remember, you're building a new you, so control that urge to start shoveling the food in as if there were no tomorrow. Remember how good you intend to look tomorrow.

A BONUS FOR YOU

If you have kept your diet for two weeks, go out to dinner with a friend and eat as prescribed but have a glass or two of dry champagne. Toast yourself. You deserve it. Then continue the diet and have another glass when the month is over. But be careful you don't get carried away.

Once you are on the maintenance plan, you can have a glass or two of champagne or white wine up to two times a week.

HOW TO BURN EXTRA CALORIES AND SPEED UP YOUR WEIGHT LOSS

1. Reduce your calorie intake. Eat less.
2. Remember that fat calories are more fattening than carbohydrate or protein calories. Be on the alert for fat and avoid it.
3. Don't go more than four hours without eating something. Have a snack. Your metabolism needs to "go into gear" at least that often to work efficiently. Also, eating lightly more often keeps you from getting too hungry, which leads to feeling as if you are starving and overeating as a result. No matter how much you tell yourself you won't overeat, if you starve yourself for ten hours, your body will take over and you **will** overeat. Do the right thing and feed your body often.
4. Try not to eat more than a snack for at least two hours before bedtime. Food is better metabolized during the day, when you can burn it off.
5. Drink lots of water.
6. Use up more energy. Do three thirty-minute aerobic sessions or more a week.
7. Increase the muscle on your body. Muscle burns calories, even while you are sleeping. The more muscles you have, the more you can eat without getting fat. (But stick to healthful low-fat, low-sugar foods.) Follow the whole body split routine and not only will you greatly increase your muscle mass but you'll find it very easy to remain trim.

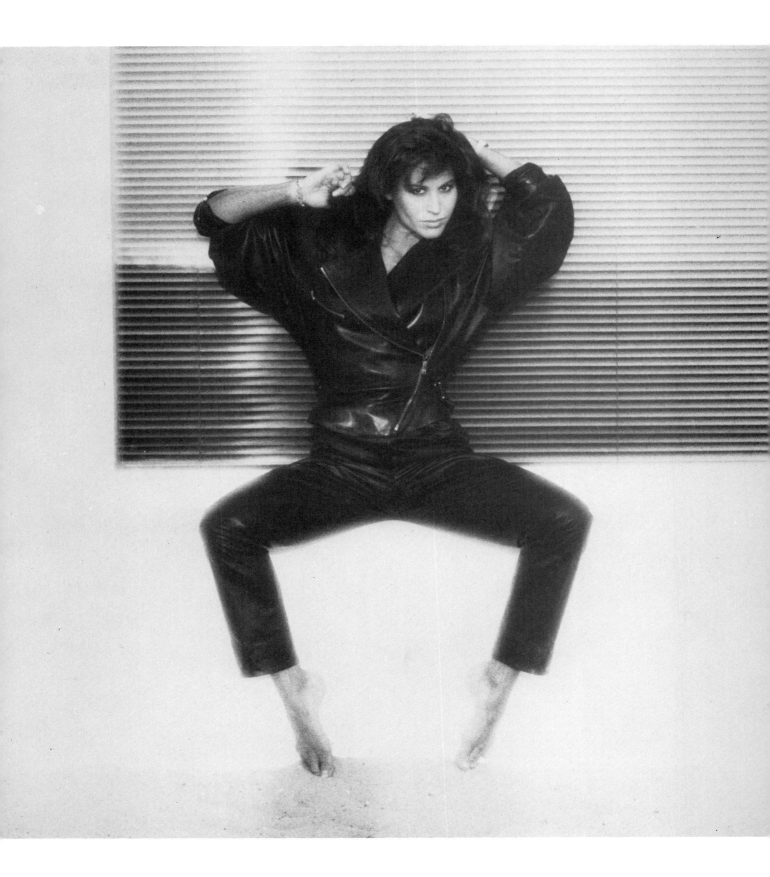

THE MAINTENANCE DIET

Continue to eat as the "diet" prescribes, but take more privileges. For example, you can have the protein pasta and tomato sauce three or four times during the week if you choose, and you can have larger portions. You can have red meat once every other week if you choose, and you can eat any and every fish on the market in place of the flounder, tuna, sole, and red snapper you've been having. You can have regular spaghetti sauce once in a while. You can eat larger portions of fresh vegetables anytime you are hungry.

One Day a Week of Eating Whatever You Choose

One day of each week, eat whatever your heart desires. If you've been craving something, go for it. Yes, even cookies or candy or ice-cream or pizza (pizza is not so bad anyway if you blot off the excess oil). Don't feel guilty. Life is meant to be enjoyed and lived in a normal fashion. You'll find that you won't stuff yourself until you can't move because you're now in control and because you love and respect your new body. You no longer live in fear of food. Food has become a normal part of life.

If you do go overboard and stuff yourself for a few days (maybe because you're going through emotional problems) you can get back on track quickly. Follow the weight-loss diet for the same number of days that you binged, then resume normal maintenance eating.

WHAT ABOUT HOLIDAYS?

Holidays are covered in your one day a week free eating. Just save your free day for a holiday. If a holiday is a season and the eating lasts for a week, then diet for one day for every one you "binged." If you ate with a vengeance for one week, diet strictly for one week, then return to normal maintenance eating.

WHAT ABOUT VACATIONS?

Just because you are on vacation doesn't mean you leave your mind at home. Sure, you can break your good eating habits from time to time, but don't make a goal of breaking every good eating habit every minute of every vacation day. You'll ruin your vacation because your body will rebel against you. You'll feel sluggish, fat, and stuffed.

Instead of stuffing yourself or eating all junk foods, why not try to stick to nutritious foods for the most part and then relish a dessert, an extra glass of champagne, or a delicious Italian dinner every so often on the vacation.

If you do throw all caution to the wind and eat and eat and eat, you know what to do: Go back on the Perfect Parts diet. If you really overdid it, diet twice as long as the binge. If you pigged out totally for two weeks, you might need to diet for a month. Fortunately, the diet itself is not so terrible, so it won't really be a punishment. Just be calm and enjoy your life. Food is only a part of life, and at least *you can control* that part.

TRAVELING

If you are traveling to a foreign country for your vacation, there's still no reason whatsoever to abandon good eating habits. Fresh fruits and vegetables can be found everywhere, and there is always a way to work around obstacles such as fried or greasy foods—just don't order them. Tell the waiter that health reasons preclude your eating them. It's true!

If you are traveling in Italy, you can enjoy plenty of pasta, which is an excellent source of complex carbohydrates. Italy is also famous for its fresh salads. I can't think of any country that doesn't have plain vegetables. For drinks, there is *always* bottled mineral water available—both carbonated and noncarbonated. The simple truth is, if there is a will—your will—then there is a way. If there is no will, and you are really looking for an excuse to blow good eating habits, then of course there is no way. Face it. It's up to you. No one can make you put something in your mouth if you don't want it put there. The choice is yours.

EXPAND THE VARIETY OF FOOD YOU EAT

It is important for both dieters and maintainers to expand the variety of healthful foods eaten. Get a copy of a nutrition book (see bibliography) and look up the names of vegetables, fruits, grains, fish, and other foods that you have never tried or that you neglect. Check to be sure the fat content is not high. If it is low, give it a try.

Don't feel obliged to always change your diet, however. You may feel comfortable with the same foods while you're dieting. If you do it's perfectly all right to stick to them, as long as you don't get so bored that you are tempted to break the good eating habits you are developing.

HOW TO MAINTAIN YOUR WEIGHT LEVEL

1. Get out of a food-focused mentality. Learn to enjoy food as a normal part of life. Get involved in the ambiance and atmosphere at mealtimes. Dine with friends often. Try different foods. Realize that you have nothing to fear in food as long as you keep your intake under control.

2. Take advantage of your free eating day. Use it to remind yourself that eating is *not* a life and death issue and that no one food can make you instantly fat.

3. Remember to maintain good eating habits during the week. It's when you cheat even a little on a day-to-day basis that fat begins to creep up on you and refuses to leave.

4. If you've binged, go on the weight loss diet for one day for every day you overindulged. Don't think of this as punishment. It's more like insurance.

5. Stay active. Activity burns calories and helps you stay trim.

6. Eat food as close to how God created it as possible—whole, raw, natural.

7. Stay in control of what you eat no matter where you are in the world or with whom. Don't let anyone tempt or intimidate you into abandoning good eating habits.

Appendix

![Summary divider bar]

SUMMARY OF THE HOME WORKOUTS

Chest Routine

1. Incline dumbbell flye
2. Flat dumbbell press
3. Cross-bench pullover
4. Hand-on-knee isometric contraction
5. Flat dumbbell flye

Back Routine

1. One-arm dumbbell bent row
2. Barbell bent row
3. Deadlift
4. Seated dumbbell back lateral
5. Straight-arm body pull

Shoulder Routine

1. Standing side lateral
2. Seated alternating dumbbell press
3. Pee Wee lateral
4. Upright row
5. Seated bent-over lateral

Biceps Routine

1. Standing alternate dumbbell curl
2. Angled simultaneous dumbbell curl
3. Standing barbell curl

Triceps Routine

1. Seated two-arm dumbbell triceps extension
2. Dumbbell kickback
3. Cross-face triceps extension

Abdominal Routine

1. Standard sit-up
2. Crunch
3. Serratus crunch
4. Knee-up leg-up combination
5. Bent-knee leg lift

Buttocks-Hip Routine

1. Standing hip hyperextension
2. Pelvic lift
3. Single-leg buttocks tightener
4. Lunge with buttocks squeeze
5. Double-leg buttocks tightener

Thigh Routine

1. Leg curl with a weight
2. Front squat
3. Lunge
4. Sissy squat
5. Bugs Bunny lunge

Calf Routine

1. One-legged calf raise
2. Calf raise—ankle rotated
3. Seated dumbbell calf raise

SUMMARY OF THE GYM WORKOUTS

Chest Routine

1. Incline dumbbell flye
2. Pec deck flye
3. Cable crossover
4. Cross-bench pullover
5. Flat dumbbell flye

Shoulder Routine

1. Standing side lateral
2. Seated alternating dumbbell press
3. Pee Wee lateral
4. Upright row
5. Seated bent-over lateral

Back Routine

1. Lat pull-down to the rear
2. Lat pull-down to the front
3. Pulley row
4. Barbell bent row
5. One-arm dumbbell row

Biceps Routine

1. Standing alternate dumbbell curl
2. Angled simultaneous dumbbell curl
3. Standing barbell curl

Triceps Routine

1. Seated two-arm dumbbell triceps extension
2. Pulley push-down
3. Cross-face triceps extension

Abdominal Routine

1. Standard sit-up
2. Crunch
3. Serratus crunch
4. Knee-up leg-up combination
5. Bent-knee leg lift

Buttocks-Hip Routine

1. Standing hip hyperextension
2. Pelvic lift
3. Single-leg buttocks tightener
4. Lunge with buttocks tightener
5. Double-leg buttocks tightener

Thigh Routine

1. Leg curl
2. Front squat
3. Lunge
4. Machine leg extension
5. Leg press

Calf Routine

1. One-legged calf raise
2. Seated calf raise
3. Standing calf machine raise

Bibliography

Hausman, Patricia, M.S. *The Calcium Bible.* New York: Rawson Associates, 1985.

Jacobson, Dr. Michael, and Bonnie F. Liebman and Gred Moyer. *Salt: The Brand Name Guide to Sodium Content.* New York: Workman Publishing Co. Inc., 1983.

Kirshbaum, John, editor. *The Nutrition Almanac, Revised Edition.* New York: McGraw-Hill Book Company, 1986.

LeGette, Bernard. *LeGette's Calorie Encyclopedia.* New York: Warner Books Inc., 1983.

McLish, Rachel. *Flex Appeal.* New York: Warner Books Inc., 1984.

Mindell, Earl. *Earl Mindell's New and Revised Vitamin Bible.* New York: Warner Books Inc., 1985.

Vedral, Joyce L. *Now or Never.* New York: Warner Books Inc., 1985.

Yanker, Gary. *Gary Yanker's Walking Workouts.* New York: Warner Books Inc., 1985.

MAGAZINES

Female Bodybuilding, 351 East 84th Street, New York, NY 10028.

Muscle and Fitness, 21100 Erwin Street, Woodland Hills, CA 91367.

Shape, 21100 Erwin Street, Woodland Hills, CA 91367.

Index

B

C

D

E

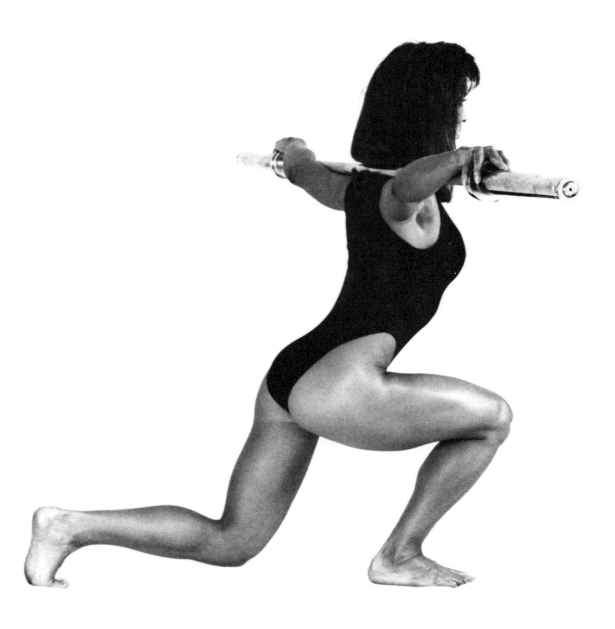

G

H

I

J

K

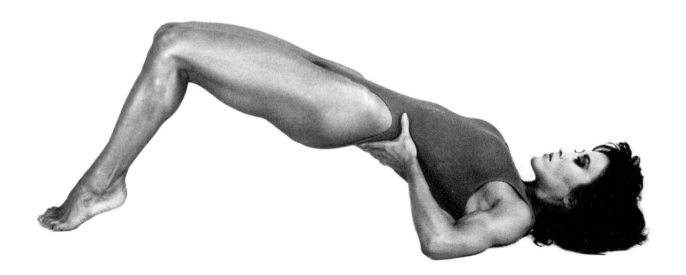

T

U

V

W

Y